OT GOALs

Occupational Therapy Goals and Objectives Associated with Learning

by Partners in GOALs

Marianne Bogdanski Aquaro, OTR

Cynthia Chauvin Gallagher, OTR

Patricia Bayruns Crocker, OTR

Ilene M. Goldkopf, OTR

Lisa A. Mulligan, OTR

Norma J. Quirk, M.S., OTR

Catherine Rainey, OTR

Michelle V. Tobias, OTR

Illustrations drawn under contract by Corwyn Zimbleman

Therapy Skill Builders
A division of
Communication Skill Builders
3830 E. Bellevue/P.O. Box 42050
Tucson, Arizona 85733/(602) 323-7500

Reproducing Pages from This Book

Many of the pages in this book can be reproduced for instructional or administrative use (not for resale). To protect your book, make a photocopy of each reproducible page. Then use that copy as a master for photocopying or other types of reproduction.

Printed and published by

Therapy Skill Builders
A division of
Communication Skill Builders ®
3830 E. Bellevue/P.O. Box 42050
Tucson, Arizona 85733/(602) 323-7500

ISBN 0-88450-544-8   Catalog No. 4244

10 9 8 7 6 5
Printed in the United States of America

For information about our audio and/or video products, write us at:
Communication Skill Builders, P.O. Box 42050, Tucson, AZ 85733.

About the Authors

Marianne Bogdanski Aquaro, OTR, received her B.S. degree in Occupational Therapy from Kean College of New Jersey in 1980. She is certified in use of the Southern California Sensory Integration Test (SCSIT) and in Neurodevelopmental Treatment (NDT). Currently she is pursuing certification in use of the Sensory Integration and Praxis Test (SIPT). Since 1980 she has practiced pediatric occupational therapy within private and public schools, hospital outpatient clinics, early intervention programs, and home-based therapy programs. She is active in program development, staff and parent education, and student programming; and she was an early advocate of classroom treatment groups and the consultative model. Ms. Aquaro was co-chair of the New Jersey Occupational Therapy Association's Pediatric Special Interest Group from 1988 to 1991.

Cynthia Chauvin Gallagher, OTR, a 1980 graduate of Kean College of New Jersey, specializes in the field of pediatric occupational therapy. She has continued her education in many areas, including attaining certification in both the Southern California Sensory Integration Test (SCSIT) and Neurodevelopmental Treatment (NDT). She was supervisor of the occupational therapy department at the Cerebral Palsy Center of Essex and West Hudson, Belleville, New Jersey; and she is the head coach for the adaptive sports program at that center. She has worked in the public schools while maintaining a part-time private practice in northern New Jersey. Areas of expertise include treatment of cerebral palsy, learning disabilities, splinting, adaptive equipment, and group work in the area of basic work and living skills.

Patricia Bayruns Crocker, OTR, received her degree in Occupational Therapy from Kean College of New Jersey. Currently she is Occupational Therapy Coordinator for Pediatrics at Associates in Physical and Occupational Therapy, Inc., a private nonprofit practice in Burlington, Vermont. She has experience in a variety of pediatric settings, including early intervention, clinic-based practice, school-based practice, and neonatal intensive care; and she is certified in Neurodevelopmental treatment (NDT). She is an associate organization faculty member in the Physical Therapy department at the University of Vermont. Currently she is pursuing a Master's degree in Education at the University of Vermont.

Ilene M. Goldkopf, OTR, is an AOTA Board Certified Pediatric Specialist. She received her degree in Occupational Therapy from Kean College of New Jersey in 1983. Ms. Goldkopf's early work experience was with severely physically challenged children at a cerebral palsy treatment center. Since 1986 she has been a partner in Skill-Builders, Inc., a private practice servicing public and private schools in central New Jersey. She has extensive experience in Sensory Integrative treatment and pediatric mental health. She is pursuing certification in use of the Sensory Integration and Praxis Test (SIPT). Ms. Goldkopf has served on the New Jersey Occupational Therapy Association's

School-Based Task Force, working toward establishing guidelines for occupational therapy practice in the New Jersey schools. She is a founding partner in Pocket Full of Therapy, a mail-order toy company specializing in toys and materials for children with learning, sensory, and/or motor difficulties.

Lisa A. Mulligan, OTR, received her degree in Occupational Therapy from Kean College of New Jersey in 1984. She has provided occupational therapy services to public and private schools throughout New Jersey. Since 1989 she has been Executive Director of Therapeutic Outreach, Inc., providing multidisciplinary therapy and Child Study Team Services for individuals from birth through age 21. She served as co-chairman of the New Jersey Occupational Therapy Association's Pediatric Special Interest Group; and was state liaison for Developmental Disabilities from 1987 through 1989. Currently she is chairman of that committee. She is a member of the New Jersey Occupational Therapy Association's School Task Force. Ms. Mulligan has written for *Channels,* the journal of the Association of Schools and Agencies for the Handicapped; and she presented a topic at the 1990 ASAH conference in Atlantic City. She is pursuing certification in use of the Sensory Integration and Praxis Test (SIPT).

Norma J. Quirk, M.S., OTR, received her B.S. degree in Elementary Education from the University of Pennsylvania; her OT certification from the Philadelphia School of Occupational Therapy; and her M.S. degree in Occupational Therapy from Temple University, Philadelphia. Ms. Quirk has worked primarily in the area of pediatrics in private and public schools. She is self-employed. In 1990 she received the New Jersey Occupational Therapy Association's Award of Merit in Pediatric Practice. Ms. Quirk believes in continuing education. She has given many presentations on the subject of occupational therapy in pediatrics. She is coauthor of *The Relationship of Learning Problems and Classroom Performance to Sensory Integration.*

Catherine Rainey, OTR, received her B.A. degree from Rutgers, the State University of New Jersey, Camden College of the Arts and Sciences; and Certification in Occupational Therapy from the University of Pennsylvania. Since 1981 she has worked in private and public school systems, providing both direct and consultation services. In collaboration with colleagues, she has authored and developed computerized occupational therapy IEP components and report-generating software that is used in 17 school districts.

Michelle V. Tobias, OTR, is an AOTA Board Certified Pediatric Specialist. She received her degree in Occupational Therapy from Quinnipiac College. Since 1976, she has worked exclusively with pediatric or developmentally disabled populations, in positions of staff therapist, consultant, and department director. She is a partner in Skill-Builders, Inc., a private occupational therapy practice in central New Jersey, servicing public and private schools and individual children. She is certified in use of the Southern California Sensory Integration Test (SCSIT) and is pursuing certification in use of the Sensory Integration Praxis Test (SIPT). She has served on the New Jersey Occupational Therapy Association's School-Based Task Force, working toward establishing guidelines for occupational therapy practice in the New Jersey schools. Ms. Tobias is a founding partner in Pocket Full of Therapy, a mail-order toy company specializing in toys and materials for children with learning, sensory, and/or motor difficulties.

CONTENTS

Goals and Objectives

Additional Material

PREFACE

OT GOALs is designed to allow the pediatric occupational therapist to efficiently complete required paperwork while integrating current theoretical frameworks and clinical experience. The wide selection of goals and objectives meets many of the diverse needs of occupational therapists working in a variety of pediatric settings. This work evolved from the authors' determination to develop more uniformity and clarity in the terminology of goals and objectives used by pediatric occupational therapists.

Throughout the writing process, no specific references have been used. The material is based on an eclectic background of theoretical frameworks including, but not limited to, normal development, sensory integration theory, and neurodevelopmental theory. This original material, created by the authors, developed from integration of professional knowledge and years of clinical experience. Each aspect of *OT GOALs* was collectively formulated by all eight authors. While this process was not the most time-efficient, it allowed us to capitalize on each author's strengths and areas of expertise.

Each goal and objective was individually analyzed for its educational relevance, ease of measurement, clarity of phrasing, and the ability to measure performance in only one isolated skill area (when possible).

OT GOALs is a valuable resource for occupational therapists working in schools and other pediatric facilities. The material is quick and efficient to use. It permits limitless application and meets the diverse needs of pediatric occupational therapists in a variety of settings.

INTRODUCTION

PURPOSE

OT GOALs is a resource for occupational therapists working with school-age children (preschool through high school). It provides an efficient method for incorporating comprehensive, measurable therapeutic goals and objectives into the child's therapy report, treatment plan, and/or Individualized Education Program (IEP). It assists administrators, teachers, other professionals, and parents in clearly communicating the target behaviors to be improved through occupational therapy. The material systematically organizes long-term goals and their accompanying objectives; and it lists qualifiers that allow for individualization. OT GOALs is not a curriculum or cookbook, and it should not be used as such.

This manual also includes information on the following:
- Guide for developing additional goals and objectives.
- Functional definitions of common terms used within OT GOALs.
- Lists of methods, strategies, materials, individuals, and types of evaluations involved in implementing goals and objectives.
- Case studies.
- Discussion, in understandable terms, of the various service delivery models of pediatric occupational therapy.

OT GOALs AND CHILD DEVELOPMENT

OT GOALs is based upon four primary domains of child development which are of specific interest to occupational therapists. Adaptive skill development, the first domain, includes long-term goals that target sensory processing, perceptual motor skills, and self-care skills. Gross motor skill development, the second area, includes long-term goals on postural control, motor planning, bilateral motor coordination, and endurance. The third domain, fine motor skill development, includes long-term goals that address upper-extremity control, fine motor and graphomotor skills, and ocular motor control. The fourth domain, personal-social skill development, includes long-term goals that focus on work behavior and task orientation and coping skills.

Skill development within and across these domains follows a common sequence and time frame. Typically, development occurs from head to toe, from proximal to distal and from gross to fine motor. However, children develop these skills at their own rates, with innate strengths and weaknesses. When delays are identified, occupational therapists must find and use the child's strengths to assist in remediating the delayed area.

OT GOALs is organized within a developmental framework. Each long-term goal area has been analyzed and broken into its subskills, reflected by the objectives. These objectives are specific, isolated skills measured through tasks and activities. The objectives are presented in a developmental sequence (as much as possible).

OT GOALs WITHIN YOUR PEDIATRIC SETTING

OT GOALs is meant to be used within a variety of pediatric settings, using a variety of occupational therapy service delivery models. These include direct service, monitoring, and consultation.

OT GOALs is based upon a working model that occupational therapy is a related service which aims to assist children to benefit from their special education programs. Thus, the long-term goals which may take a greater length of time to achieve are educationally based. If the educational base is inappropriate for your occupational therapy setting, long-term goals may be adjusted, new ones may be formulated, or other objectives substituted.

TREATMENT DELIVERY MODELS AND *OT GOALs*

OT GOALs is designed to meet the diverse demands of a pediatric therapist and the various models of service delivery that may be offered. These include the direct therapy, monitoring, and consultative models.

DIRECT THERAPY SERVICE

In this service model, individual or small groups of children are seen in occupational therapy once to several times a week. The student's baseline status is determined through an occupational therapy assessment of strengths and weaknesses. Long-term goals and objectives are established based upon the baseline status and parent-teacher consultation. The occupational therapist then implements a treatment plan to address the goal areas. Progress and effectiveness of therapy are evaluated periodically by the occupational therapist.

MONITORING

In the monitoring model, the occupational therapist provides the student, teacher, and/or parents with specific treatment ideas and activities as well as basic information on the student's areas of strength and weakness. As in the direct therapy service model, the goals and objectives are established based upon the student's baseline status. A treatment plan is developed by the occupational therapist and then implemented by a predetermined other. The student is reassessed by the occupational therapist at established intervals and the program is adjusted accordingly. This service model may be used:

1. In conjunction with direct therapy service.

2. As a transition for students previously receiving direct therapy services.

3. For students who are considered at risk for developmental delays which may interfere with their educational performance.

4. For students who may benefit from therapeutic input in specific areas of weakness more frequently within their educational and home environments.

CONSULTATION

Occupational therapy consultation is usually requested to address a specific problem or to make broad recommendations or changes. The consultative information is designed to have ongoing impact within the student's educational and home environments. The student may or may not previously have received occupational therapy services. Baseline information may be obtained through observation, screening, and/or report. Problem solving may then occur to determine the appropriate strategy, compensation, adaptive technique, and/or device needed. The student's goal areas may have been established by the IEP team with or without occupational therapy input. Occupational therapy consultation may contribute to the attainment of those goals. Consultation occurs on an "as needed basis," varying anywhere from once a week to once a year.

OT GOALs AND THE LAW

The Education of All Handicapped Children Act (EHA) of 1975 (PL 94-142) and its regulations (34 Code of Federal Regulations [CFR] 34, Part 300.1) have four main purposes:

"1. To insure that all handicapped children have available to them a free appropriate public education which includes special education and related services to meet their unique needs" (as outlined in the individualized education program).

"2. To insure that the rights of handicapped children and their parents are protected.

"3. To assist states and localities to provide for the education of all handicapped children.

"4. To assess and insure the effectiveness of efforts to educate those children."

The CFR 34 (300.13) further defines and describes the purpose of related services as being "the transportation and such developmental, corrective and other supportive services as are required to assist a handicapped child to benefit from Special Education. . . ." Occupational therapy is listed as a related service; and it is partially defined as:

"1. Improving, developing, or restoring functions impaired or lost through illness, injury, or deprivation;

"2. Improving ability to perform tasks for independent functioning when functions are impaired or lost;

"3. Preventing, through early intervention, initial or further impairment or loss of function."

P.L. 99-457 of 1986 was an amendment to the Education of All Handicapped Children Act (EHA) of 1975 (P.L. 94-142). This amendment extended eligibility for special education services for children three to five years old.

The Individuals with Disabilities Education Act (IDEA) of 1990 (P.L. 101-476) amended both P.L. 94-142 and 99-457 (EHA). P.L. 101-476 continues to guarantee the provisions under these two laws. The major provisions added under IDEA include but are not limited to:

1. Changing the name of "Education of All Handicapped Children Act (EHA)" to "Individuals with Disabilities Education Act (IDEA)."

2. Changing the term "handicapped" to "disabled" and using language that emphasizes the individual instead of the disability.

3. Adding transition services from school to community as a requirement of the individualized education program (IEP).

4. Adding new disabilities to the list of conditions eligible for special education services.

The IEP continues to be a major provision required by this education legislation. A main purpose of *OT GOALs* is to assist occupational therapists in efficiently completing their portion of the IEP using qualitative measurable goals and objectives.

In addition to the previously cited educational legislation, several other legislative acts impact on the delivery of education and therapeutic services to individuals with disabilities.

Section 504 of the Rehabilitation Act of 1973 (P.L. 93-112) was enacted to prevent discrimination against individuals with disabilities who are in programs receiving federal funding. This act created the Architectural and Transportation Barriers Compliance Board which addresses issues surrounding access to public buildings and transportation. This act is significant to therapists working with children and young adults by emphasizing services which eliminate or minimize physical barriers to education, employment, and vocational opportunities and community activities.

The Americans with Disabilities Act (ADA) of 1990 (P.L. 101-336) emphasizes the integration of all individuals with disabilities into the social and physical "mainstream of American life" (National Mental Health Association, 1990, p. 1).

Title I of this amendment places emphasis on employment and vocation of individuals with disabilities. Title II, much like Section 504, addresses access to public services, programs, and facilities, regardless of whether they receive federal funds. Title III of ADA enforces agencies, excluding private residences and religious facilities. Title IV guarantees access to telecommunications by individuals with "speech or hearing" disabilities. Throughout these titles, ADA stipulates that "reasonable accommodations" be made and promotes the use of "auxiliary aids" to access services and programs.

Both Section 504 and ADA are pertinent to *OT GOALs* in that many of the goals and objectives stated in this book measure those occupational therapy services which will promote the integration of individuals with disabilities and enable institutions and community programs and activities to comply with existing legislation.

This section covered the primary legislation which relates to the use of *OT GOALs*. However, interpretation of this cited legislation varies among states. As a result, special education policies and the occupational therapist's role within each state may vary. Therapists are encouraged to review thoroughly this federal legislation, as well as state legislation, and to contact their State Department of Education and local special education departments for further definition and interpretation of the law.

National Mental Health Association. 1990. *Legislative Summary Series, Americans with Disabilities Act of 1990 (Public Law 101-336)*. Alexandria, VA.: National Mental Health Association.

THE IEP PROCESS

Each child who is eligible for special services is required by federal law to have a written, parent-signed Individualized Education Plan (IEP). This plan includes the child's goals and objectives for the year. The IEP is to be reviewed each year and a new one formulated.

School districts vary in their procedures for implementing this process. The role of the occupational therapist within this process also varies.

MODELS OF OCCUPATIONAL THERAPY INPUT

There are several common models of school procedures that state what is expected of team members. Each model begins with individual disciplines completing their appropriate assessments to establish the student's baseline status.

Model 1. Team members meet to discuss findings. Goals and objectives are then established separately for each discipline.

Model 2. Team members meet, discuss findings, and establish overall long-term goals. Team members in the individual disciplines then separately determine short-term objectives to address each of the established long-term goals.

Model 3. Team members meet and discuss findings. All long-term goals and objectives are established together.

Model 4. Team members meet and discuss findings. Long-term goals are established together. The formulation of objectives is then assigned as appropriate.

Model 5. In some situations, appropriateness, final approval, and inclusion of specific goals and objectives may be determined by a case manager, parents, the overall team, or the core team.

PARENTAL INVOLVEMENT

The Code of Federal Regulations addresses parental involvement by describing the parent's role, rights, and procedural safeguards. The Local Education Agency (LEA) must include procedures to ensure the participation of and consultation with parents or guardians of all children with disabilities. The procedural safeguards primarily protect the rights of both the children and their parents. Under section 438 of the General Educational Provisions Act and Part 99 of Family Education Rights and Privacy Act of 1974, the parents have the right of confidentiality of information concerning their children. Parents have the right to prior notice that the child needs to be evaluated, the right to consent to evaluations and individualized education programs, the right to a copy of the IEP, and the right to participate in the IEP meeting. The law also guarantees access rights of parents to inspect and review any educational records relating to their children. This access must be within 45 days of the request. Parents have a right to a response from the facility to reasonable requests for explanations and interpretations of records and/or copies of those records, and the right to a due-process hearing when there is disagreement between the parents and the public agency regarding the appropriate program for the child. Parents also have the right to an independent educational evaluation of their child at school expense. Parents have the right to request amendments of the child's records. Parental consent must be obtained before personally identifiable information is either disclosed or used for any purpose other than meeting an IEP requirement.

The Code of Federal Regulations defines the parental role at the IEP meeting as follows: "Parents of a child with disability are expected to be equal participants, along with school personnel, in developing, reviewing, and revising the child's IEP. This is an active role in which parents (1) participate in the discussion about the child's need for special education and related services, and (2) join with the other participants in deciding what services the agency will provide to the child" (p. 84). The LEA must take steps to ensure that at least one parent is present at meetings (IEP conferences and annual reviews). The agency must notify parents early and schedule meetings at a mutually agreed-upon time and place. If neither parent can attend, the public agency shall use other methods to ensure parent participation, including individual or conference telephone calls. The IEP meeting can be held without parents, but school representatives must document attempts to involve parents. The school must take "whatever action is necessary to ensure that the parent understands the proceedings at a meeting." For example, the school must arrange for an interpreter for parents with hearing impairments or who are non-English speaking.

Related service also "includes school health services, social work services in schools, and parent counseling and training" (p. 14). "Parent counseling and training is further defined to mean assisting parents in understanding the special needs of their child and providing parents with information about child development" (p. 15). Occupational therapy input is invaluable in this aspect of parent education in addition to direct provision of service to the child. Further, the law stipulates that agencies include personnel development systems which provide inservice training and dissemination of significant information to both staff and parents.

DURATION AND FREQUENCY OF TREATMENT

"Must the IEP specify the amount of services or may it simply list the services to be provided?"

"The amount of services to be provided must be stated in the IEP, so that the level of the agency's commitment of resources will be clear to parents and other IEP team members. The amount of time to be committed to each of the various services to be provided must be (1) appropriate to that specific service, and (2) stated in the IEP in a manner that is clear to all who are involved in both the development and implementation of the IEP. Changes in the amount of services listed in the IEP cannot be made without holding another IEP meeting or an addendum made in writing. However, as long as there is no change in the overall amount, some adjustments in scheduling the services should be possible (based on the professional judgment of the service provider) without holding another IEP meeting. Note: The parents should be notified whenever this occurs" (Code of Federal Regulations, p. 90).

STRATEGIES AND METHODS

"Objectives in IEPs are different from those used in instructional plans, primarily in the amount of detail they provide. . . Classroom instructional plans generally include details not required in an IEP, such as the specific methods, activities, and materials (e.g., use of flash cards) that will be used in accomplishing the objectives" (Code of Federal Regulations, p. 88).

"The IEP is not intended to be detailed enough to be used as an instructional plan. The IEP, through its goals and objectives, (1) sets the general direction to be taken by those who will implement the IEP, and (2) serves as the basis for developing a detailed instructional plan for the child" (Code of Federal Regulations, p. 89).

According to the Code of Federal Regulations (Education 34, Parts 300-399), methods and strategies are not a required part of the IEP. However, they are formulated as a part of the child's instructional guide. In New Jersey, many districts attach the instructional guide to the IEP.

HOW TO WRITE AN INSTRUCTIONAL GUIDE FOR AN IEP

The instructional guide provides the parent, teacher, and others with an idea of how the child's program will be implemented, and how each person working with that child can reinforce goal areas. As with the goals and objectives, the instructional guide should be written in collaboration with those involved in the child's life.

See page 13 for a reproducible Instructional Guide form. Many schools and programs use this instructional guide format, while others may use a different format; yet the essential information is the same. If your school or clinic does not require this guide, you might still decide to include one because it enhances the carryover of intervention into the child's daily routine.

The *Goal* column is self-explanatory. Each specific long-term goal area being addressed is listed in this column. See pages 21-22 and 33-36 for the long-term goals included in this book.

The *Method* column indicates how the intervention will be provided to implement each goal area. This does not include frequency and duration; that information is listed elsewhere in the child's IEP or formal evaluation report. This section may include the roles of other individuals who will be involved in implementing a goal and may not be inclusive of the occupational therapist's role in working with the child. See page 14 for a list of methods which are used in this book.

The *Strategy* column describes the specific types of intervention to be used to achieve the designated goal area(s). These strategies may include a particular teaching or therapeutic approach, a grading or adaptation to an activity, and other approaches. See pages 15-16 for a list of strategies used in this book. These strategies highlight only the primary modes of intervention which will be provided; it cannot list every type of strategy that will be used with the child.

The *Material* column lists therapeutic and educational equipment and toys which may be used to reinforce goal areas. It does not list a specific toy or equipment; rather, it describes possible categories of toys and equipment which may be appropriate for the goal area. Thus, it helps individuals generalize the types of appropriate materials that can be used with the child. See pages 16-17 for a list of materials referred to in this book.

The *Who* column lists individuals who will be involved in implementing each goal area. In this way, use of the resources that are available to the child is maximized. See page 17 for a list of individuals referred to in this book.

The *Evaluation* column describes how the mastery of each goal area will be measured and evaluated. This is not limited to formal evaluations only. It may involve parental or teacher report of performance in the goal areas. We chose not to list specific evaluation tools, which may vary depending on the clinic or school system and/or area of the country. See page 18 for a list of evaluations which are used in this book.

INSTRUCTIONAL GUIDE

Goals and Objectives

Name _____

Date _____

Goal	Method	Strategy	Material	Who	Evaluation	Comments

METHODS*

1. Individual occupational therapy intervention

2. Occupational therapy large-group intervention

3. Occupational therapy small-group intervention

4. Occupational therapy monitoring

5. Occupational therapy consultation with appropriate staff members

6. Occupational therapy consultation with the classroom teacher

7. Occupational therapy consultation with the special education teacher

8. Occupational therapy consultation with the child's classroom parapro-fessional

9. Occupational therapy consultation with the physical educator

10. Occupational therapy consultation with the adaptive physical educator

11. Occupational therapy consultation with the speech-language pathologist

12. Occupational therapy consultation with the physical therapist

13. Co-treatment sessions with the physical therapist

14. Co-treatment sessions with the speech-language pathologist

15. Team teaching with the classroom teacher

16. Team teaching with the physical education teacher

17. Team teaching with adaptive physical education

18. Home programming suggestions

19. Parent/Caregiver intervention

20. Classroom teacher intervention

21. Special educator/Teacher intervention

22. Physical educator intervention

23. Adaptive physical educator intervention

24. Physical therapy intervention

25. Speech-language therapy intervention

*Other methods may be added as needed.

STRATEGIES*

1. Provide minimal/moderate/maximum assistance.

2. Provide verbal cues as needed.

3. Provide demonstration as needed.

4. Provide hand-over-hand assistance.

5. Utilize therapeutic preparatory techniques with ongoing use of these techniques as needed to facilitate adaptive responses.

6. Present gross motor activities in developmental sequence.

7. Present fine motor activities in developmental sequence.

8. Adapt gross motor activities as needed.

9. Grade gross motor activities as needed.

10. Adapt fine motor activities as needed.

11. Grade fine motor activities as needed.

12. Teach compensatory techniques.

13. Provide practice and repetition to reinforce skill development.

14. Adjust the child's positioning to improve performance.

15. Provide positive reinforcement.

16. Guide the child through the motions of a fine motor activity to provide tactile/proprioceptive and kinesthetic feedback.

17. Guide the child through the motions of a gross motor task to provide tactile/proprioceptive and kinesthetic feedback.

18. Provide a multisensory approach as required.

19. Require the child to specify an organizational plan before the task is implemented.

20. Enhance the child's participation through high-interest activities.

21. Provide minimal/moderate/maximum ongoing structure for task completion.

22. Provide decreasing structure for task completion.

23. Provide a work space with minimal/moderate/maximum distractions.

24. Utilize experimental learning techniques.

25. Provide written instructions.

26. Provide adaptive equipment as needed.

27. Utilize forward chaining techniques.

(continued)

*Other strategies may be added as needed.

28. Utilize backward chaining techniques.

29. Utilize activities with increasing number of steps or sequences.

30. Utilize multistep activities.

31. Utilize upper extremity weight-bearing activities.

32. Present visual-motor activities in developmental sequence.

MATERIALS*

1. Suspended equipment (netswings, platform swing, etc.)

2. Scooterboard(s)

3. Tactile stimulatory activities (shaving cream, finger paint, etc.)

4. Toys/materials requiring resistive grasp and squeeze (clay, water pistols, tongs, tweezers, etc.)

5. Toys/materials with very small pieces (pegs, bead stringing, etc.)

6. Playground equipment

7. Adaptive equipment

8. Puzzles

9. Books

10. Toys incorporating size concepts

11. Toys incorporating shape concepts

12. Stringing toys (beads, macaroni, sewing cards, spools, etc.)

13. Cut-and-paste activities

14. Coloring activities

15. Tracing activities

16. Balls in a variety of sizes

17. Beanbag activities

18. Target games

19. Pretend or symbolic play activities

20. Dress-up costumes

21. Computer games

22. Specialized computer software

23. Board games

24. Riding toys

*Other materials may be added as needed.

25. Toys requiring twisting and untwisting

26. Obstacle courses

27. Hidden-picture games

28. Paper-pencil mazes

29. Dot-to-dot sheets

30. Painting with assorted paintbrushes

31. Clay dough activities

32. Therapeutic exercises

33. Small/medium/large therapy ball

34. Small/medium/large bolster

35. Small/medium/large wedge

36. Balance-beam activities

37. Scissors activities

38. General classroom tools (hole punch, ruler, paper clips)

39. Scented materials

WHO*

1. Occupational therapist

2. Physical therapist

3. Speech-language pathologist

4. Parent/Caregiver

5. Classroom teacher

6. Special education teacher

7. Physical education teacher

8. Adaptive physical educator

9. Paraprofessional/Teacher's aide

10. Student

*Others may be added as needed.

EVALUATIONS*

1. Occupational therapist clinical observations

2. Classroom teacher observations

3. Special education teacher observations

4. Physical education teacher observations

5. Adaptive physical educator observations

6. Speech-language pathologist observations

7. Parent/Caregiver observations

8. Child/Student report

9. Fine motor evaluation

10. Gross motor evaluation

11. Visual-motor evaluation

12. Visual perception evaluation

13. Goniometric evaluation

14. Manual muscle testing

15. Muscle-tone testing

16. Sensory testing

17. Developmental evaluation

18. Standardized testing

---

*Other evaluations may be added as needed.

GOALS AND OBJECTIVES

OT GOALs

Eleven long-term goal areas are identified in this book. A list of all long-term goals and 55 general objective areas is provided as a quick reference on pages 33-36, along with 648 specific objectives.

Briefly stated, the long-term goal areas are:

Pages 41-48   LTG 1   Sensory processing—Objectives dealing with accommodation, awareness, tolerance, discrimination, and organization of touch, movement, and auditory and olfactory stimuli.

Pages 49-54   LTG 2   Postural control—Objectives dealing with co-contraction, protective responses, and balance and equilibrium reactions.

Pages 55-75   LTG 3   Upper-extremity control and fine motor skills—Objectives dealing with reach, release, grasp-and-pinch patterns, dominance, lateralization, midrange control, and grading of force, strength, isolated finger control, in-hand manipulation, scissor use, and range of motion.

Pages 77-84   LTG 4   Motor planning—Objectives dealing with proprioception/kinesthesis, ideation, and planning and execution of motor tasks.

Pages 85-91   LTG 5   Bilateral motor coordination—Objectives dealing with crossing of midline; and movements which are symmetrical, asymmetrical, and reciprocal.

Pages 93-98   LTG 6   Ocular motor control—Objectives dealing with visual skills of focusing, tracking, scanning, and localization.

Pages 99-111   LTG 7   Perceptual motor skills—Objectives dealing with body awareness, spatial awareness, and the visual perceptual skills of sequencing, figure-ground discrimination, and closure.

Pages 113-120   LTG 8   Written communication—Objectives dealing with prewriting and writing, using classroom tools, and keyboarding skills.

The objectives are designed to allow a great deal of flexibility and individualization for each client. Within each objective, there are choices to be made by the therapist, based upon the child's current skill level and expected level of improvement. These choices are referred to as "qualifiers." They are designed to expedite and individualize the therapist's formulation of objectives. They also allow the objectives to be graded in terms of skill level difficulty. See pages 37-38 for a listing of all qualifiers. For ease in using *OT GOALs*, however, relevant qualifiers also are listed on the left-hand side of the individual objectives pages. These lists contain only those qualifiers which apply to the objectives on that page.

HOW TO USE *OT GOALs*

Using *OT GOALs* is a simple process.

1. The first step is to assess the child, determining strengths and weaknesses and identifying areas of need.

2. Select long-term goal areas corresponding to identified areas of need. (For example, if a child is found to have difficulty with fine motor skills and midline crossing, then long-term goals 3 and 5 would be selected.) See pages 21-22 and 33-36 for the long-term goals referred to in this book.

3. Once long-term goals are selected, review the general objectives listed under each long-term goal. Select those objectives which will most efficiently measure progress toward the long-term goals. See pages 33-36 for a list of objective areas referred to in this book.

4. Specific objectives are listed following each long-term and general goal. Select specific objectives which will most efficiently produce progress toward the long-term goals and general objectives. Several specific objectives may be used simultaneously.

5. Have the child attempt the selected specific objectives, establishing baselines of performance. Once baselines are determined, each objective can be tailored to the individual child by selecting specific qualifiers and appropriate means of measurement. See pages 37-38 for a list of all qualifiers referred to in this book; or use the quick reference list of qualifiers provided on each objectives page.

6. If the goals and objectives provided in *OT GOALs* do not appear to meet the needs of a specific child, the therapist may need to create customized goals. To assist in writing original goals, see "Guide for Developing Customized Goals and Objectives" (pages 24-25).

7. Appropriate and behavioral long-term goals and objectives now have been set. Documentation of the chosen goals and objectives can be accomplished by hand-writing them in detail; or you can use one of the *OT GOALs* worksheets (pages 28 or 30) to speed the process. Refer to pages 26-27 for instructions on how to use the worksheets, and see the samples on pages 29 and 31.

GUIDE FOR DEVELOPING CUSTOMIZED GOALS AND OBJECTIVES

While 55 general and 648 specific objectives are provided in *OT GOALs*, there may be times when totally customized, original objectives are needed. The following guide is provided to assist therapists in producing effective behavioral objectives.

Long-term goals identify the *general area* to be addressed, as well as explain the functional importance of that area. For many children, a long-term goal may remain appropriate for an extended period of time.

Objectives are specific *isolated skills*, measured by tasks and activities, which will assist in the acquisition and development of the long-term goal.

By definition, behavioral objectives must be observable and measurable, and any therapist must be able to reproduce them. They must be written in understandable terms that promote teacher-parent comprehension. Each objective should measure, as much as possible, only one isolated skill component.

Objectives should be attainable within one year. Several objectives may be used simultaneously.

Each objective should include an answer to the following five questions:
1. *Who?* Who is to perform the skill?

2. *What?* What action is being performed, or what skill is being measured?

3. *How?* What material is being used to measure the skill? How is the material or skill being qualified? (See page 40 for a list of materials referred to in this book, and pages 37-38 for a list of the qualifiers referred to here.)

4. *Where?* In what position or location is the skill being performed?

5. *When?* How frequently or how many times is the skill being performed? (See page 39 for a list of ratios and percentages.)

After writing the objective, review it for clarity and ease of understanding. Avoid the use of professional jargon and terms which may not be easily understood by others. Check the objective for reproducibility; that is, whether another therapist or tester will clearly understand what is being tested and how to accomplish the objective.

The following chart shows construction of two customized objectives.

Sample Customized Objectives

Objective 1. The child will use hands symmetrically to propel a scooterboard forward while prone, 10 times.

Who?	What?	How?	Where?	When?
What action is being performed, or what skill is being measured?	*What action is being performed, or what skill is being measured?*	*a. What material is being used?* *b. How is the material or skill being qualified?*	*In what position or location is the skill being performed?*	*How frequently or how many times is the skill being performed?*
The child	will use hands symmetrically to propel	a scooterboard forward	while prone	10 times

Objective 2. The child will hold and sort three coins one at a time with one hand, 7 out of 10 times.

Who?	What?	How?	Where?	When?
What action is being performed?	*What action is being performed?*	*a. What material is being used?* *b. How is the material or skill being qualified?*	*In what position or location is the skill being performed?*	*How frequently or how many times is the skill being performed?*
The child	will hold and sort	three coins one at a time	with one hand	7 out of 10 times

THE *OT GOALs* WORKSHEETS

The *OT GOALs* worksheets are meant to be timesaving tools in the process of organizing, denoting, and customizing the long-term goals and objectives chosen for each client. They allow the therapist to do this quickly by using only a few letters and numbers. Later, this information can easily be transposed (by a secretary or by the therapist) onto the final document (for example, the IEP or treatment plan) by referring to the pages and sections of *OT GOALs* indicated on the worksheet. This eliminates the need for the therapist to hand-write each goal and objective in its entirety, only to rewrite or type it on the final document later. *The worksheets themselves are* not *meant to be placed into the final documentation!* Therapists also may find the worksheets helpful as a quick reference on those goals and objectives which have been selected for a client, or to denote improvements and changes over time.

Worksheet A (see page 28) is designed to record only long-term goals and objectives, with their appropriate qualifiers. This type of goal writing may be most appropriate for treatment plans.

Worksheet B (see page 30) can be used when additional information is required. The form provides space for indicating goal and objective methods, strategies, materials, evaluators, and types of evaluations. This type of goal writing may be more appropriate for IEPs, since these areas usually are referred to in the Instructional Guide section of the IEP.

Choose the worksheet that best meets your needs and is most appropriate for your school's requirements. Please note that the number of goals and objectives needed for each client may and should vary, depending upon the client's needs and school requirements. Worksheet A contains space for listing 10 goals and objectives, and Worksheet B has space for 6 listings. These numbers are not intended to indicate that all should be used or that more cannot be used. Reproduce the worksheets and use as many for each client as you deem necessary.

HOW TO USE WORKSHEETS A AND B

(As you read this section, it is important to refer to the sample worksheets provided on pages 29 and 31.)

1. Choose Worksheet A or B, according to your needs.

2. Select the first long-term goal area to be addressed. (See pages 21-22 for a quick reference to all long-term goals included in *OT GOALs.*) On the worksheet, write the number of that long-term goal in the space after the first LTG. (For example, if the goal is to improve arm and hand control, select LTG 3.)

3. Select the first general objective area to be addressed. (See pages 33-36 for a quick reference to all general objective areas included in *OT GOALs*.) On the worksheet, write the letter of that general objective in the space after OBJ. (For example, if arm strength and stability are needed, select letter G under Long-Term Goal 3.)

4. Refer to the pages indicated next to each general objective area listed on pages 33-36. (For example, the listing for Objective G indicates pages 64-65.) Turn to those pages, and review the list of specific objectives. Select the objective that is most appropriate for the client. These specific objectives are numbered. Write the corresponding number on the worksheet. (In the examples on pages 29 and 31, we used #9, "using an overhand method to throw.")

5. Within the specific objective, one or more blanks must be filled in. These are referred to as "qualifiers." The qualifier category is named. (In #9, for example, "Type of Ball" must be filled in.) On the Goals and Objectives page, choices are listed in the left-hand column. Locate the appropriate category, and choose the qualifier that is most appropriate for the client. Write the qualifier (or its corresponding letter) in the space after "Qualifiers" on the worksheet. (In the example, in the "Type of Ball" category, we selected "a. volley" and wrote "a." in the "Qualifiers" space on the worksheet.)

In some objectives (such as #9, which we are using in our example), a number must be determined. There are *no* number qualifiers listed to the left; the therapist must determine the number that is appropriate for the client. (In the example, we decided to require the volleyball to be thrown a distance of five feet, and we wrote "5" in the "Qualifiers" space.)

If you are using Worksheet A, repeat the process of selecting goals and objectives until all therapist-determined areas are completed.

If you are using Worksheet B, a few additional steps are needed.
6. The methods of how the goal will be addressed must be listed. See page 14 for a list of methods. Select one or more, and place the corresponding numbers after "Methods" on the worksheet. (In the example, we selected #1, "Individual occupational therapy intervention," and #6, "Occupational therapy consultation with the classroom teacher." On the worksheet, we wrote "1, 6" after "Methods.")

7. Select "Strategies" (see pages 15-16), and write the corresponding number on the worksheet.

8. Select "Materials" (see pages 16-17), and write the corresponding number on the worksheet.

9. Select who will be responsible for assessing and implementing the goal (see "Who," page 17), and write the corresponding number on the worksheet.

10. Select "Evaluations," or how the goal will be assessed (see page 18), and write the corresponding number on the worksheet.

Repeat steps 1-10 until all therapist-determined areas are completed.

OT GOALs WORKSHEET A

Occupational Therapy Goals and Objectives 19_____-19_____

Name: _____ Therapist: _____

Date: _____ District: _____

Code:
LTG = Long-Term Goal
OBJ = Objective
# = Number of Objective
Qualifiers = (Fill in from Qualifiers list)

Page _____   LTG _____; OBJ _____; # _____; Qualifiers _____

Page _____   LTG _____; OBJ _____; # _____; Qualifiers _____

Page _____   LTG _____; OBJ _____; # _____; Qualifiers _____

Page _____   LTG _____; OBJ _____; # _____; Qualifiers _____

Page _____   LTG _____; OBJ _____; # _____; Qualifiers _____

Page _____   LTG _____; OBJ _____; # _____; Qualifiers _____

Page _____   LTG _____; OBJ _____; # _____; Qualifiers _____

Page _____   LTG _____; OBJ _____; # _____; Qualifiers _____

Page _____   LTG _____; OBJ _____; # _____; Qualifiers _____

Page _____   LTG _____; OBJ _____; # _____; Qualifiers _____

OT GOALs WORKSHEET A

Occupational Therapy Goals and Objectives 19_93_ -19_94_

Name: _Sam Gee_   Therapist: _L. Jones, OTR_

Date: _9-26-93_   District: _Sunnyslope_

Code:
LTG = Long-Term Goal
OBJ = Objective
# = Number of Objective
Qualifiers = (Fill in from Qualifiers list)

Page _65_   LTG _3_ ; OBJ _1_ ; # _9_____ ; Qualifiers _a, 5_____

Page _____   LTG ____; OBJ ____; # _____ ; Qualifiers _____

Page _____   LTG ____; OBJ ____; # _____ ; Qualifiers _____

Page _____   LTG ____; OBJ ____; # _____ ; Qualifiers _____

Page _____   LTG ____; OBJ ____; # _____ ; Qualifiers _____

Page _____   LTG ____; OBJ ____; # _____ ; Qualifiers _____

Page _____   LTG ____; OBJ ____; # _____ ; Qualifiers _____

Page _____   LTG ____; OBJ ____; # _____ ; Qualifiers _____

Page _____   LTG ____; OBJ ____; # _____ ; Qualifiers _____

Page _____   LTG ____; OBJ ____; # _____ ; Qualifiers _____

Page _____   LTG ____; OBJ ____; # _____ ; Qualifiers _____

OT GOALs WORKSHEET B

Occupational Therapy Goals and Objectives 19_____-19_____

Name: _____ Therapist: _____

Date: _____ District: _____

Code:
LTG = Long-Term Goal   # = Number of Objective
OBJ = Objective   Qualifiers = (Fill in from Qualifiers list)

Page _____ LTG _____; OBJ _____; # _____; Qualifiers _____;

Methods _____; Strategies _____; Materials _____;

Who _____; Evaluations _____

Page _____ LTG _____; OBJ _____; # _____; Qualifiers _____;

Methods _____; Strategies _____; Materials _____;

Who _____; Evaluations _____

Page _____ LTG _____; OBJ _____; # _____; Qualifiers _____;

Methods _____; Strategies _____; Materials _____;

Who _____; Evaluations _____

Page _____ LTG _____; OBJ _____; # _____; Qualifiers _____;

Methods _____; Strategies _____; Materials _____;

Who _____; Evaluations _____

Page _____ LTG _____; OBJ _____; # _____; Qualifiers _____;

Methods _____; Strategies _____; Materials _____;

Who _____; Evaluations _____

Page _____ LTG _____; OBJ _____; # _____; Qualifiers _____;

Methods _____; Strategies _____; Materials _____;

Who _____; Evaluations _____

Sample
OT GOALs WORKSHEET B

Occupational Therapy Goals and Objectives 19 *93* -19 *94*

Name: *Sam Gee*   Therapist: *R. Jones, OTR*

Date: *9-26-93*   District: *Sunnyslope*

Code:
LTG = Long-Term Goal   # = Number of Objective
OBJ = Objective   Qualifiers = (Fill in from Qualifiers list)

Page *65* LTG *3* ; OBJ *2* ; # *9* ; Qualifiers *a, 5* ;

Methods *1, 6* ; Strategies *17* ; Materials *16* ;

Who *1* ; Evaluations *1, 4*

Page _____ LTG _____ ; OBJ _____ ; # _____ ; Qualifiers _____ ;

Methods _____ ; Strategies _____ ; Materials _____ ;

Who _____ ; Evaluations _____

Page _____ LTG _____ ; OBJ _____ ; # _____ ; Qualifiers _____ ;

Methods _____ ; Strategies _____ ; Materials _____ ;

Who _____ ; Evaluations _____

Page _____ LTG _____ ; OBJ _____ ; # _____ ; Qualifiers _____ ;

Methods _____ ; Strategies _____ ; Materials _____ ;

Who _____ ; Evaluations _____

Page _____ LTG _____ ; OBJ _____ ; # _____ ; Qualifiers _____ ;

Methods _____ ; Strategies _____ ; Materials _____ ;

Who _____ ; Evaluations _____

Page _____ LTG _____ ; OBJ _____ ; # _____ ; Qualifiers _____ ;

Methods _____ ; Strategies _____ ; Materials _____ ;

Who _____ ; Evaluations _____

QUICK REFERENCE LIST OF LONG-TERM GOALS AND GENERAL OBJECTIVES

QUALIFIERS USED THROUGHOUT *OT GOALs*

Sizes
a. small
b. medium
c. large
d. ___-inch

Accuracy
a. ___ inches
b. ___ feet
c. only ___ errors
d. within a ___-inch space
e. ___ degrees
f. ___ deviation

Hand/Foot Usage
a. preferred
b. nonpreferred
c. bilateral
d. both
e. right
f. left
g. unilateral
h. symmetrical(ly)
i. asymmetrical(ly)
j. reciprocal
k. alternate(ly)(ing)
l. stabilizer
m. gross assist
n. functional assist
o. active assist
p. one
q. (any combination of bilateral, unilateral, symmetrical, asymmetrical, reciprocal alternates)

Duration
a. seconds
b. minutes
c. repetitions

Grasps
a. lateral
b. three-point
c. two-point
d. tip-tip
e. opposition

Plane
a. horizontal
b. vertical
c. diagonal
d. circular
e. rotary
f. pendular
g. linear
h. forward
i. backward
j. sideways
k. forward, backward, and sideways
l. multidirectional

Graphomotor
a. manuscript
b. cursive
c. upper
d. lower
e. A to Z

Dressing
a. coats/sweaters
b. hat
c. gloves/mittens
d. boots
e. shoes
f. socks
g. button-down smock/shirt
h. pullover smock/shirt
i. belt
j. braces/orthotics
k. clothes

Fasteners
a. large buttons
b. small buttons
c. separating zipper
d. nonseparating zipper
e. snaps
f. buckle
g. Velcro®

Spatial Concepts
a. in/out of
b. on/off of
c. under/over
d. in front of/ in back of
e. next to/beside
f. through
g. up/down
h. behind

Velcro® is a registered trademark of Velcro U.S.A., Inc.

Quality

a. without hyperextension
b. with wrist held in neutral or extended position
c. without overflow
d. without fixing
e. with rhythm
f. with fluidity
g. using mature patterns
h. grading
i. directed
j. timing

Strength
(Manual Muscle Test)

a. ___ lbs.
b. fair
c. fair +
d. good -
e. good
f. good +
g. normal

Body Movements

a. flexion
b. extension
c. abduction
d. adduction
e. external rotation
f. internal rotation
g. ulnar deviation
h. radial deviation
i. pronation/pronated
j. supination/supinated
k. opposition/opposed
l. neutral
m. (any combination of above)

Type of Ball

a. volley
b. beach
c. ___-inch playground
d. ___-inch therapy
e. hard
f. tennis
g. basket
h. ___-inch foam
i. base
j. medicine
k. racket
l. Wiffle®
m. cage

Classroom Tools

a. standard classroom scissors
b. squeeze or easy-grip scissors
c. adapted scissors
d. sharp scissors
e. ruler
f. stapler
g. compass
h. hole punch
i. pencil sharpener
j. one-inch blade scissors
k. tape dispenser

Type of Assistance

a. assistance
b. supervision
c. guidance
d. prompt
e. demonstration
f. cues
g. in functional activities
h. independently
i. with gravity (assisted)
j. gravity eliminated
k. against gravity
l. with __ facilitation to ___
m. with adapted devices
n. passive
o. active
p. adaptive techniques
q. (any combination of above)

Body Parts

a. chest
b. abdomen
c. knees
d. hips
e. shoulder
f. ankle
g. thigh
h. thumb
i. index finger
j. long/middle finger
k. ring finger
l. little (pinky) finger

Shapes

a. vertical line
b. horizontal line
c. circle
d. crossed lines
e. X
f. square
g. triangle
h. vertical diamond
i. horizontal diamond

School-Related
Activities

a. physical education
b. playground
c. classroom
d. fine motor
e. gross motor
f. postural
g. desk top
h. (any specific activity of your choice)

Degree of Assistance

a. minimum(ly)
b. moderate(ly)
c. maximum(ly)
d. verbal
e. hand-over-hand
f. physical
g. tactile
h. auditory
i. visual
j. no
k. (any combination of above)

Wiffle® is a registered trademark of The Wiffle Ball, Inc., Shelton, CT.

PERCENTAGE CONVERSION TABLE

Throughout the manual, every objective is measurable and utilizes either ratios (such as 3 out of 4 times) or percentages (such as 75%). The following grid may be useful in completing the objectives. It states frequently used ratios and their equivalents in percentages.

Ratio	Percentage
1 out of 2	50%
3 out of 5	60%
2 out of 3	67%
3 out of 4	75%
4 out of 5	80%
17 out of 20	85%
6 out of 7	86%
9 out of 10	90%
(1 out of 1) 5 out of 5	100%

SPECIFIC MATERIALS
MENTIONED IN *OT GOALs*

1/2-gallon container
1/2-pint milk carton
balance beam
balancing blocks
balloons
balls
beads (pop type)
beads (stringing type)
beanbags
belt
bike (foot-driven)
bike (hand-driven)
bike (mobile)
bike (stationary)
blocks (balancing)
blocks (one-inch)
bolster
books
boots
bottle (finger-pump
    spray type)
bottle (squeeze type)
bottle (trigger spray
    type)
bowl and spoon
braces
car (foot-driven)
car (hand-driven)
car (mobile)
car (stationary)
cards, color
cards, deck of 52
cards, pattern (with
    parquetry blocks)
cards, picture
cards, shape
chair
chalkboard and chalk
clay
clay dough
clothespins
coat
color cards
computer keyboard
containers (used as
    targets)

cotton balls
crayons
cubes (one-inch)
cup/glass
deck of cards
desk/work surface
dominoes
doors
eraser (chalkboard)
eraser (pencil)
finger paints
finger-pump spray
    bottle
fork
glass/cup
gloves/mittens
glue
glue bottle
hole punch (one-hole)
jacket
jar with lid
jump rope
knife
laces
linking monkeys
linking shapes
marbles
mat
milk carton
mittens/gloves
monkeys (linking)
multiplane track (for
    cars or marbles)
netswing
nuts and bolts
one-inch blocks/cubes
paddle/racquet
paper
parquetry blocks with
    pattern cards
pegboard
pegs of various sizes
pencil
pencil sharpener
picture cards
pop beads

putty (color coded)
puzzles
racquet/paddle
ring toss/horseshoes
rope
rubber bands
ruler
sand
scissor tongs
scissors
scooterboard
screws with nuts
shape cards
shapes, linking
shirt (button type)
shirt (pullover type)
shoes with laces
small objects
socks
spoon
spray bottle (finger-
    pump type)
spray bottle (trigger
    type)
straws
streamers
swing
tactile objects (sand,
    clay, glue, finger
    paints)
tape and tape recorder
therapy ball
tissues
toilet
tongs
trigger spray bottle
tweezers
typewriter
washcloth
water faucet
water gun
Wiffle® ball
wind-up toy
work surface/desk
zipper garment

Wiffle® is a registered trademark of The Wiffle Ball, Inc., Shelton, CT.

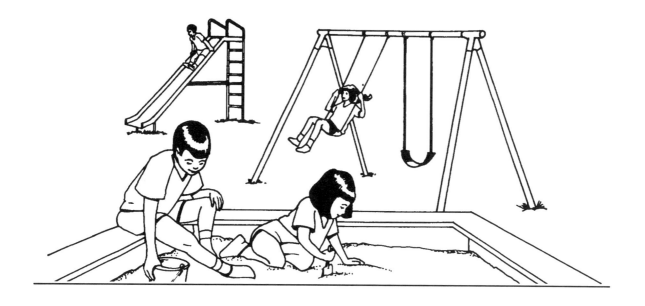

LONG-TERM GOAL
1

To improve ability to use sensory information to understand and effectively interact with people and objects in school and home environments.

Long-Term Goal 1

To improve ability to use sensory information to understand and effectively interact with people and objects in school and home environments.

Objective A

To demonstrate improved accommodation to touch sensations, _____ (*child's name*) will:

*1. Accept anticipated touch during a group activity, ___ out of ___ times.

*2. Accept hands-on assistance during task performance without showing signs of discomfort, for ___ seconds.

3. Accept unexpected touch without behavioral overreactions, ___% of the time.

*4. Sit or stand in a group without behavioral overreactions, ___% of the time.

*5. Participate in various tactile activities (such as sand, clay, glue, finger painting, food preparation, and finger feeding) without behavioral overreactions, ___% of the time.

*6. Participate in school activities without engaging in nonpurposeful bumping, banging, and crashing behaviors, ___% of the time.

7. Recognize familiar small objects placed in ___ (*Hand/Foot Usage*) hand, using sense of touch only, ___% of the time.

8. Recognize shapes or lines "drawn" on back of ___ (*Hand/Foot Usage*) hand, when vision was occluded, ___ out of ___ times.

9. Indicate which finger was touched on back of ___ (*Hand/Foot Usage*) hand, when vision was occluded, ___ out of ___ times.

Customized objectives:

* These objectives are skills to be observed within the classroom setting. They may be especially useful in the total team-generated IEP models.

School-Related Activities
a. physical education
b. playground
c. classroom
d. fine motor
e. gross motor
f. postural
g. desk top
h. (any specific activity of your choice)

Plane
a. horizontal
b. vertical
c. diagonal
d. circular
e. rotary
f. pendular
g. linear
h. forward
i. backward
j. sideways
k. forward, backward, and sideways
l. multidirectional

NOTES

Long-Term Goal 1

To improve ability to use sensory information to understand and effectively interact with people and objects in school and home environments.

Objective B

To demonstrate improved accommodation to movement sensations, _____ (child's name) will:

1. Initiate participation in a ___ (School-Related Activity) activity (slides, climbing, etc.) involving self-imposed movement on an immobile surface in a ___ (Plane) plane for ___ minutes.

2. Initiate participation in a ___ (School-Related Activity) activity involving self-imposed movement on a movable surface in a ___ (Plane) plane for ___ minutes.

3. Participate in a functional activity involving imposed movement in a ___ (Plane) plane for ___ minutes.

4. Participate in a ___ (School-Related Activity) activity involving imposed movement on a movable surface in a ___ (Plane) plane for ___ minutes.

5. Maintain participation in group movement activities involving changing planes, directions, and rhythms for ___ minutes, ___ out of ___ sessions.

Customized objectives:

Size
a. small
b. medium
c. large
d. ____-inch

NOTES

Long-Term Goal 1

To improve ability to use sensory information to understand and effectively interact with people and objects in school and home environments.

Objective C

To demonstrate improved awareness and discrimination of touch sensations, _____ (*child's name*) will:

1. Find ___ (*number*) ___ (*Size*) objects hidden in a container of textured material (rice, sand, beans), within ___ minutes, with vision occluded.

2. Differentiate between safe and dangerous touching of objects, ___% of the time.

3. Differentiate between necessary and unnecessary touching of objects and/or people, ___% of the time.

*4. Inhibit unnecessary touching of objects and/or people for ___ minutes.

5. Point to the place on fingers that was touched lightly when vision was occluded, within ___ centimeters of accuracy.

6. Point to the place on arm or hand that was touched lightly when vision was occluded, within ___ centimeters of accuracy.

7. Feel shape placed in hand, with vision occluded, and identify corresponding object, given ___ (*number*) choices, ___ out of ___ times.

8. Feel shape placed in hand, with vision occluded, and identify corresponding picture given, ___ (*number*) choices, ___ out of ___ times.

9. Identify familiar, common objects placed in hand, with vision occluded, ___ out of ___ times.

10. Match ___ (*number*) out of ___ (*number*) shapes, with vision occluded.

11. Match ___ (*number*) out of ___ (*number*) items by size, with vision occluded.

12. Match ___ (*number*) out of ___ (*number*) textures, with vision occluded.

13. Point to the picture of a shape that matches the one "drawn" on hand while vision was occluded, ___ out of ___ times.

14. Feel, with vision occluded, among many shapes and find the one previously designated, ___ out of ___ times.

Customized objectives:

* These objectives are skills to be observed within the classroom setting. They may be especially useful in the total team-generated IEP models.

Long-Term Goal 1

To improve ability to use sensory information to understand and effectively interact with people and objects in school and home environments.

Objective D

To demonstrate improved organization of auditory input _____ (*child's name*) will:

*1. Consistently stop activity and/or look up when appropriate (for example, in response to teacher, fire alarm, intercom).

*2. Remain seated and calm in a classroom while sounds (such as class bell, car, airplane, or buzzer, etc.) occur, ___% of the time.

*3. Continuously engage in an activity for ___ minutes, with auditory distractions.

*4. Discriminate between relevant and irrelevant auditory stimuli as evidenced by the ability to attend in the classroom, gym, and auditorium for ___ minutes, in the presence of auditory distractions.

5. Discriminate volume of sound by accurately describing it as loud, soft, etc., ___ out of ___ times.

*6. Identify the location of sound, ___ out of ___ times.

*7. Identify and attend to sounds and warnings of potential harm within environment, ___% of the time.

*8. Follow ___ (*number*) -step verbal directions without use of visual cues or gestures, ___% of the time.

9. Accurately repeat a ___ (*number*) -step direction.

Customized objectives:

* These objectives are skills to be observed within the classroom setting. They may be especially useful in the total team-generated IEP models.

Long-Term Goal 1

To improve ability to use sensory information to understand and effectively interact with people and objects in school and home environments.

Objective E

To demonstrate improved awareness and tolerance of olfactory (smell) stimuli, _____ (*child's name*) will:

*1. Alert or respond when a scent has been introduced, ___% of the time.

2. Identify and attend to potentially harmful odors within the environment, ___% of the time.

*3. Continue working in the presence of environmental odors (for example, food, cleaning agents, perfume) ___% of the time.

*4. Engage in activities involving a scent (for example, playing with clay dough, cooking, gluing) for ___ minutes, without adverse reactions or undue distress.

Customized objectives:

---

* These objectives are skills to be observed within the classroom setting. They may be especially useful in the total team-generated IEP models.

Degree of Assistance
a. minimum(ly)
b. moderate(ly)
c. maximum(ly)
d. verbal
e. hand-over-hand
f. physical
g. tactile
h. auditory
i. visual
j. no
k. (any combination of above)

Type of Assistance
a. assistance
b. supervision
c. guidance
d. prompt
e. demonstration
f. cues
g. in functional activities
h. independently
i. with gravity (assisted)
j. gravity eliminated
k. against gravity
l. with ___ facilitation to ___
m. with adapted devices
n. passive
o. active
p. adaptive techniques
q. (any combination of above)

NOTES

Long-Term Goal 1

To improve ability to use sensory information to understand and effectively interact with people and objects in school and home environments.

Objective F

To demonstrate improved ability to calm self and inhibit nonpurposeful movements, _____(*child's name*) will:

*1. With ___ (*Degree of Assistance*) ___ (*Type of Assistance*) participate in a stationary activity, with less than ___ (*number*) extraneous movements, within ___ minutes.

*2. Participate in a stationary activity, with less than ___ (*number*) extraneous movements, within ___ minutes.

*3. Perform a desk-top activity for ___ minutes, with less than ___ (*number*) movement breaks.

*4. Participate in a motor activity, with less than ___ (*number*) extraneous movements, within ___ minutes.

Customized objectives:

* These objectives are skills to be observed within the classroom setting. They may be especially useful in the total team-generated IEP models.

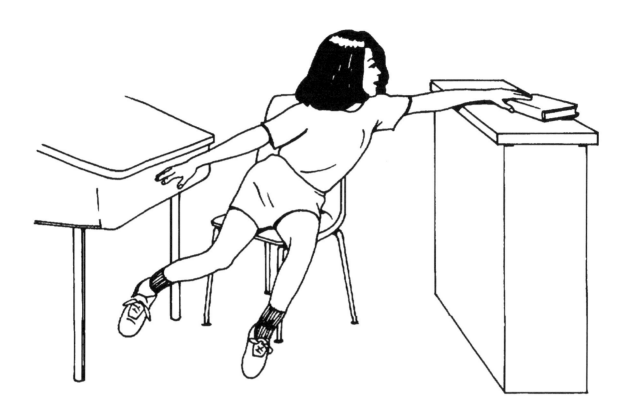

LONG-TERM GOAL

2

To improve postural control to provide a stable base of support needed to facilitate better hand use for manipulation of classroom materials, posture while working or playing, and mobility in school and home environments.

QUALIFIERS

Body Parts
a. chest
b. abdomen
c. knees
d. hips
e. shoulder
f. ankle
g. thigh
h. thumb
i. index finger
j. long/middle finger
k. ring finger
l. little (pinky) finger

NOTES

Long-Term Goal 2

To improve postural control to provide a stable base of support needed to facilitate better hand use for manipulation of classroom materials, posture while working or playing, and mobility in school and home environments.

Objective A

To demonstrate improved balance between flexor and extensor musculature (cocontraction), _____ (*child's name*) will:

1. Maintain a lifted and extended posture of the head and upper body from a prone position (on stomach), for ___ seconds.

2. Maintain a lifted and extended posture of the legs, with the legs straight and the thighs slightly off the floor, from a prone position (on stomach), for ___ seconds.

3. Maintain a lifted and extended posture of the entire body, from a prone position (on stomach), for ___ seconds.

4. Maintain an extended trunk and head position with arms outstretched to the sides for ___ seconds, while lifted with support provided at the ___ (*Body Parts*) and the legs wrapped around therapist's waist.

5. Maintain a lifted and curled position of the neck and shoulders, with arms crossed over chest, from a supine position (on back), for ___ seconds.

6. Maintain a lifted position of the knees into the chest from a supine position (on back), for ___ seconds.

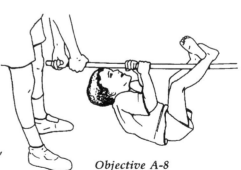

Objective A-4

7. Maintain a lifted and curled posture of the entire body, with arms crossed over chest, from a supine position (on back), for ___ seconds.

8. While lifted, maintain grasp on a dowel held parallel to body when supine, with legs hooked over dowel and head maintained approximately ___ inches from dowel, for ___ seconds.

Objective A-8

9. Maintain a lifted and extended posture of the head, upper body, and legs while propelling a scooterboard, in prone position (on stomach), for a distance of ___ feet.

(continued)

51

Long-Term Goal 2, Objective A (continued)

10. Hold onto a bolster with arms and legs wrapped around it and with back positioned toward ceiling while bolster is tilted at an angle of 45 degrees from the floor, for ___ seconds.

11. Hold onto a bolster with arms and legs wrapped around it and with back toward floor while bolster is tilted at an angle of 45 degrees from the floor, for ___ seconds.

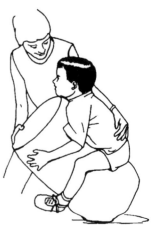

*12. Maintain a functional sitting posture with upright head and trunk, hips at 90 degrees, and feet flat on the floor, without support from arms, during a fine motor activity, for ___ minutes.

Objective A-10

*13. Maintain a functional sitting posture with upright head and trunk, hips at 90 degrees, and feet flat on the floor, without support from arms, during classroom fine motor activities, ___% of the time.

Customized objectives:

---

* These objectives are skills to be observed within the classroom setting. They may be especially useful in the total team-generated IEP models.

QUALIFIERS

Plane
a. horizontal
b. vertical
c. diagonal
d. circular
e. rotary
f. pendular
g. linear
h. forward
i. backward
j. sideways
k. forward, backward, and sideways
l. multidirectional

NOTES

Long-Term Goal 2

To improve postural control to provide a stable base of support needed to facilitate better hand use for manipulation of classroom materials, posture while working or playing, and mobility in school and home environments.

Objective B

To improve spontaneous use of protective responses, _____ (*child's name*) will:

1. Demonstrate a protective response (including extension of the arms) when moved quickly forward while prone (on stomach) over a large ball, ___ out of ___ times.

*2. Demonstrate a protective response (including extension of the arms) when shifted off balance in a ___ *(Plane)* direction while sitting on the floor, ___ out of ___ times.

3. Demonstrate a protective response (including extension of the arms) when shifted off balance in a ___ *(Plane)* direction while sitting in a chair, ___ out of ___ times.

Customized objectives:

---

* These objectives are skills to be observed within the classroom setting. They may be especially useful in the total team-generated IEP models.

Hand/Foot Usage
  a. preferred
  b. nonpreferred
  e. right
  f. left

NOTES

Long-Term Goal 2

To improve postural control to provide a stable base of support needed to facilitate better hand use for manipulation of classroom materials, posture while working or playing, and mobility in school and home environments.

Objective C

To improve balance/equilibrium reactions, _____ (*child's name*) will:

1. Respond with trunk, arm, and leg movement of one side when shifted to the opposite side, while kneeling, ___ out of ___ times.

2. Respond with trunk, arm, and leg movement of one side when shifted to the opposite side, while half kneeling, ___ out of ___ times.

*3. Respond with trunk, arm, and leg movement of one side when shifted to the opposite side, while standing, ___ out of ___ times.

*4. Maintain sitting in a chair, without holding on, when shifted off balance in any plane, ___ out of ___ times.

5. Maintain half-kneeling when shifted off balance in all planes, ___ out of ___ times.

6. Maintain standing when shifted off balance in all planes, ___ out of ___ times.

*7. Maintain posture or position during functional activities while in sitting, for ___ minutes.

*8. Maintain posture or position during functional activities while in standing, for ___ minutes.

*9. Adapt posture as challenged by playground activities and/or equipment, ___% of the time.

10. Stand still on ___ (*Hand/Foot Usage*) foot, with eyes open and arms crossed over chest, for ___ seconds.

11. Stand still on ___ (*Hand/Foot Usage*) foot, with eyes closed and arms crossed over chest, for ___ seconds.

12. Walk on a ___-inch wide balance beam for ___ feet, ___ out of ___ times.

13. Walk on a ___-inch wide balance beam using a heel-toe pattern for ___ feet, ___ out of ___ times.

Customized objectives:

---

* These objectives are skills to be observed within the classroom setting. They may be especially useful in the total team-generated IEP models.

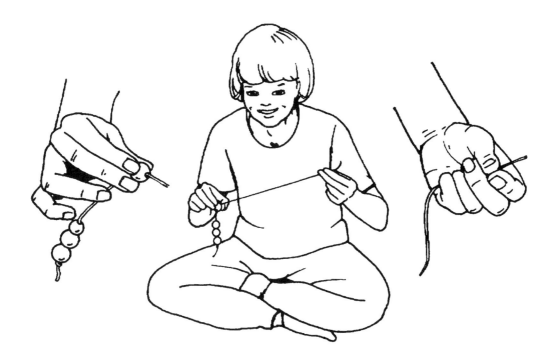

LONG-TERM GOAL
3

To improve functional shoulder, arm, and hand control for greater success with fine motor tasks and classroom and home manipulatives.

Hand/Foot Usage
  c. bilateral
  g. unilateral

Body Movements
  i. pronation/pronated
  j. supination/supinated
  l. neutral

NOTES

Long-Term Goal 3

To improve functional shoulder, arm, and hand control for greater success with fine motor tasks and classroom and home manipulatives.

Objective A

To demonstrate purposeful and accurate reach toward objects, _____(child's name) will:

1. Use a visually directed ___ (Hand/Foot Usage) approach in any direction, ___ out of ___ times.

2. Use an auditorially directed ___ (Hand/Foot Usage) approach in any direction, ___ out of ___ times.

3. Use an appropriate ___ (Body Movement) forearm reach pattern, ___ out of ___ times.

4. Use an appropriate reach pattern, ___ out of ___ times.

Customized objectives:

Long-Term Goal 3

To improve functional shoulder, arm, and hand control for greater success with fine motor tasks and classroom and home manipulatives.

Objective B

To demonstrate appropriate release patterns, _____(*child's name*) will:

1. Purposefully use surface to assist in the release of an object, ___ out of ___ times.

2. Utilize controlled release of an object above a ___ *(Size)* container with wrist extension, ___ out of ___ times.

3. Release a small object from a pincer grasp with wrist extension, ___ out of ___ times.

4. Tower ___ *(number)* ___-inch blocks, ___ out of ___ times.

Customized objectives:

Long-Term Goal 3

To improve functional shoulder, arm, and hand control for greater success with fine motor tasks and classroom and home manipulatives.

Objective C

To demonstrate appropriate grasp or pinch pattern,_____
(*child's name*) will:

*1. Use voluntary flexion of fingers only against surface to grasp (rake) object(s), ___ out of ___ times.

*2. Use flexion of fingers against object pressed into palm with thumb adduction to grasp (palmar) object(s), ___ out of ___ times.

*3. Use flexion of fingers against object pressed into thumb side of palm with thumb opposition to grasp (radial palmar) object(s), ___ out of ___ times.

*4. Hold object between opposed thumb and pads of fingers with no palm involvement (radial digital grasp), ___ out of ___ times.

*5. Hold object between adducted thumb and side of index finger (lateral pinch), ___ out of ___ times.

*6. Hold object between thumb and index finger (inferior pincer grasp), ___ out of ___ times.

*7. Hold object between pads of opposed thumb, index and long/middle fingers (three-point grasp), ___ out of ___ times.

*8. Hold object between pads of opposed thumb and index finger with thumb and finger slightly flexed (neat pincer), ___ out of ___ times.

*9. Hold object between tips of opposed thumb and index finger (fine pincer), ___ out of ___ times.

*10. Use static tripod grasp when writing with a pencil, ___% of the time.

*11. Use dynamic tripod grasp when writing with a pencil, ___% of the time.

*12. Grasp presented objects using a functional or compensatory pattern, ___ out of ___ times.

*13. Use adaptive equipment to grasp presented objects, ___ out of ___ times.

Customized objectives:

* These objectives are skills to be observed within the classroom setting. They may be especially useful in the total team-generated IEP models.

QUALIFIERS

Hand/Foot Usage
a. preferred
e. right
f. left

School-Related Activities
a. physical education
b. playground
c. classroom
d. fine motor
e. gross motor
f. postural
g. desk top
h. (any specific activity of your choice)

Degree of Assistance
a. minimum(ly)
b. moderate(ly)
c. maximum(ly)
d. verbal
e. hand-over-hand
f. physical
g. tactile
h. auditory
i. visual
j. no
k. (any combination of above)

Type of Assistance
a. assistance
b. supervision
c. guidance
d. prompt
e. demonstration
f. cues
g. in functional activities
h. independently
i. with gravity (assisted)
j. gravity eliminated
k. against gravity
l. with ___ facilitation to ___
m. with adapted devices
n. passive
o. active
p. adaptive techniques
q. (any combination of above)

Long-Term Goal 3

To improve functional shoulder, arm, and hand control for greater success with fine motor tasks and classroom and home manipulatives.

Objective D

To demonstrate a hand preference or dominance, _____ (*child's name*) will:

1. Reach for and grasp objects with ___ (*Hand/Foot Usage*) hand, ___ out of ___ times.

2. Reach for an object and manipulate it with the same hand, ___% of the time.

3. With ___ (*Degree of Assistance*) ___ (*Type of Assistance*), initiate and complete an activity consistently using the same hand, ___% of the time.

4. With ___ (*Degree of Assistance*) ___ (*Type of Assistance*), use nonpreferred hand only as an assisting hand during bimanual tasks, ___% of the time.

*5. Use drawing/writing implement with only ___ (*Hand/Foot Usage*) hand, ___% of the time.

*6. With ___ (*Degree of Assistance*) ___ (*Type of Assistance*), initiate and complete a ___ (*School-Related Activity*) using ___ (*Hand/Foot Usage*) hand, ___% of the time.

7. Perform most activities using a ___ (*Hand/Foot Usage*) dominant pattern, ___% of the time.

*8. Cut with scissors with dominant hand while other hand assists by turning paper, ___% of the time.

*9. Hold ruler in place with assisting hand while making pencil line with dominant hand, ___ out of ___ times.

*10. With preferred hand, successfully use a spoon with ___ (*Degree of Assistance*) ___ (*Type of Assistance*), ___% of the time.

*11. With preferred hand, successfully use a fork with ___ (*Degree of Assistance*) ___ (*Type of Assistance*), ___% of the time.

Customized objectives:

---

* These objectives are skills to be observed within the classroom setting. They may be especially useful in the total team-generated IEP models.

Long-Term Goal 3

To improve functional shoulder, arm, and hand control for greater success with fine motor tasks and classroom and home manipulatives.

Objective E

To demonstrate internalized awareness of the difference between two sides of the body, _____(child's name) will:

1. Indicate which hand was weighted during an activity, within ___ (number) seconds after completing task, ___ out of ___ times.

*2. Identify right and left body sides/hands on self, within ___ (number) seconds, ___ out of ___ times.

*3. Identify right and left sides of an object, within ___ (number) seconds, ___ out of ___ times.

*4. Identify right and left sides of paper, within ___ (number) seconds, ___ out of ___ times.

5. Move to the ___ (Hand/Foot Usage) direction, within ___ (number) seconds when verbally cued, ___ out of ___ times.

*6. Identify right and left body parts during a motor activity such as "Hokey Pokey," ___ out of ___ times.

*7. Identify the right or left sides of the paper, ___% of the time.

*8. Form horizontal line on paper moving from left to right, with verbal cues only, ___ out of ___ times.

*9. Form left-to-right and right-to-left diagonal lines on paper, with verbal cues only, ___ out of ___ times.

Customized objectives:

---

* These objectives are skills to be observed within the classroom setting. They may be especially useful in the total team-generated IEP models.

Fraction
    1/4-inch
    1/2-inch
    3/4-inch
    1 inch (2 inches, etc.)

NOTES

Long-Term Goal 3

To improve functional shoulder, arm, and hand control for greater success with fine motor tasks and classroom and home manipulatives.

Objective F

To demonstrate arm midrange control/grading of movement, using appropriate force and accuracy, in order to perform physical education, art, and classroom activities with control and precision, _____ (*child's name*) will:

1. Throw a beanbag into a ___-inch container from ___ (*number*) feet away, ___ out of ___ times.

2. Throw a ___-inch ball into a ___-inch container or hoop from ___ (*number*) feet away, ___ out of ___ times.

3. Toss rings or horseshoes to hit a game stick from ___ (*number*) feet away, ___ out of ___ times.

4. Throw any ball against a wall from a distance of ___ (*number*) feet with appropriate force for it to return safely, within ___ (*number*) attempts.

5. Consecutively hit a balloon to eye level with hand while maintaining elbow at side, ___ out of ___ times.

6. Place and balance a beanbag on a paddle or racket, toss it up approximately ___ (*number*) inches, and recatch it using only the paddle, ___ out of ___ times.

7. Place ___ (*number*) sized pegs into a board without undershooting or overshooting the holes, ___ out of ___ times.

*8. Color a simple ___-inch shape, staying within ___ (*Fraction*) of the boundary.

*9. Stack ___ (*number*) one-inch cubes without arm resting on table.

10. Hook ___ (*number*) monkey or shape pieces together to form a suspended chain.

11. Stack ___ (*number*) pieces of a balancing block game without arm resting on the table.

*12. Accurately pour liquid from a 1/2-pint milk container into a small plastic drinking cup, ___% of the time.

13. Accurately pour liquid from a 1/2-gallon container into an 8-ounce glass, ___% of the time.

(continued)

---

* These objectives are skills to be observed within the classroom setting. They may be especially useful in the total team-generated IEP models.

QUALIFIERS

Fraction
1/4-inch
1/2-inch
3/4-inch
1 inch (2 inches, etc.)

Degree of Assistance
a. minimum(ly)
b. moderate(ly)
c. maximum(ly)
d. verbal
e. hand-over-hand
f. physical
g. tactile
h. auditory
i. visual
j. no
k. (any combination of above)

Type of Assistance
a. assistance
b. supervision
c. guidance
d. prompt
e. demonstration
f. cues
g. in functional activities
h. independently
i. with gravity (assisted)
j. gravity eliminated
k. against gravity
l. with ___ facilitation to ___
m. with adapted devices
n. passive
o. active
p. adaptive techniques
q. (any combination of above)

14. Rest ___ *(number)* marbles on holes of a large pegboard without jarring any other marbles while working.

15. Place the second triangular parquetry piece onto a square or diamond outline without displacing the first piece, within ___ *(number)* attempts.

*16. Place four one-inch cubes together to form a large square without displacing the other cubes while working, within ___ *(number)* attempts.

*17. Place parquetry blocks onto ___ *(number)*-block design card without displacing previously placed blocks more than ___ times.

18. Stand ___ *(number)* dominoes vertically, approximately one inch apart, to form a chain without any falling.

*19. Press computer or electric typewriter keys with appropriate pressure to type only one character for each touch, ___ out of ___ times.

*20. Effectively remove from and/or insert tape recorder cassette in ___ *(number)* attempt(s).

*21. Maintain adequate pressure on glue bottle to evenly cover a ___ *(Fraction)*-long line.

*22. Squeeze and release a standard glue bottle to form ___ *(number)* small glue dots, within ___ *(number)* attempts.

*23. Grasp objects (for example, homework paper, sandwich) without crushing, ___% of the time.

*24. Successfully use a spoon with ___ *(Degree of Assistance)* ___ *(Type of Assistance)*, ___% of the time.

Customized objectives:

---

* These objectives are skills to be observed within the classroom setting. They may be especially useful in the total team-generated IEP models.

Long-Term Goal 3

To improve functional shoulder, arm, and hand control for greater success with fine motor tasks and classroom and home manipulatives.

Objective G

To demonstrate improved arm strength and stability, which are needed as a foundation for controlled movement, _____(child's name) will:

1. Reach with alternating hands while propped on forearms in prone (on stomach), for ___ (number) minutes (for example, while turning pages of a book/assembling puzzles).

2. With ___ (Degree of Assistance) ___ (Type of Assistance), reach with free hand while supported on other forearm in side-sit position, for ___ (number) minutes on each side (for example, while stacking blocks/ playing board game).

3. With ___ (Degree of Assistance) ___ (Type of Assistance), reach with free hand across midline while supported on an extended arm in side-sit position, for ___ (number) minutes on each side (for example, while assembling puzzles/playing with pegboard).

4. With ___ (Degree of Assistance) ___ (Type of Assistance), reach with alternating hands while maintaining quadriped (hands and knees), for ___ (number) minutes (for example, while rolling a ball).

5. Reach with alternating hands while prone on extended arms over a ___ (Size) bolster (diameter larger than child's arm length) which is placed under the ___ (Body Part), for ___ (number) minutes.

6. Reach with alternating hands while prone on extended arms over a ___ (Size) ball (diameter larger than child's arm length) which is placed under the ___ (Body Part), for ___ (number) minutes.

7. With ___ (Degree of Assistance) ___ (Type of Assistance), reach with alternating hands across midline while leaning back on externally rotated and extended arms in a long-sitting position, for ___ (number) minutes (for example, while throwing beanbags at a target).

8. Push off from a wall using hands while prone (on stomach) on a scooterboard, ending with hands at least ___ (number) feet from the wall, ___ times.

(continued)

* These objectives are skills to be observed within the classroom setting. They may be especially useful in the total team-generated IEP models.

*9. Use an overhand method to throw a ___ *(Type of Ball)* ball for a distance of ___ *(number)* feet.

10. Propel a scooterboard while prone (on stomach) for ___ *(number)* feet, using hands only.

11. Wheelbarrow-walk for a distance of ___ *(number)* feet, with support provided at the ___ *(Body Part)*.

*12. Participate in a ___ *(School-Related Activity)* activity, for ___ *(number)* minutes, with ___ *(number)* rest periods.

13. Pull along a rope using a hand-over-hand pattern, while prone (on stomach) on a scooterboard, for a distance of ___ *(number)* feet.

14. Pull along a ___ *(number)*-foot rope, using a hand-over-hand pattern, while prone (on stomach) in a netswing.

*15. Independently ___ *(push/pull)* open a school lavatory and/or exit door.

*16. Pull a wagon which has ___ *(number)* child(ren) in it for a distance of ___ *(number)* feet.

*17. Push a classroom desk a distance of ___ *(number)* feet.

18. Move self forward and back ___ *(number)* times while sitting tailor-fashion on a scooter and ___ *(pushing/pulling)* while holding onto adult's hands.

*19. Carry mealtime items with ___ *(Degree of Assistance)* ___ *(Type of Assistance)*, ___% of the time.

*20. Pour liquids without spilling with ___ *(Degree of Assistance)* ___ *(Type of Assistance)*, ___% of the time.

Customized objectives:

* These objectives are skills to be observed within the classroom setting. They may be especially useful in the total team-generated IEP models.

Body Parts
a. chest
b. abdomen
c. knees
d. hips
e. shoulder
f. ankle
g. thigh
h. thumb
i. index finger
j. long/middle finger
k. ring finger
l. little (pinky) finger

NOTES

Long-Term Goal 3

To improve functional shoulder, arm, and hand control for greater success with fine motor tasks and classroom and home manipulatives.

Objective H

To demonstrate isolated finger control, _____(child's name) will:

*1. Extend each finger consecutively as in counting, ___% of the time.

*2. Point or poke with index finger, keeping all other fingers flexed, ___% of the time.

*3. Trace desired form with one extended finger, ___ out of ___ times.

*4. Trace desired form with one extended finger keeping all others flexed, ___ out of ___ times.

5. Abduct and adduct extended fingers, ___ (number) times, within ___ (number) seconds.

6. Consistently touch thumb to each finger one at a time, as in finger circles.

7. Consecutively touch thumb to each fingertip one at a time (opposition), ___ out of ___ times.

8. Flick marble with thumb and ___ (Body Part) finger, within ___ (number) attempts.

9. Flick marble with each finger consecutively, within ___ (number) attempts.

*10. Depress intended keyboard characters with only extended ___ (Body Part) finger, ___ out of ___ times.

*11. Reach keyboard characters with an individual finger while maintaining other fingers in home-row position, ___% of the time.

*12. Use appropriate fingers to produce recognizable signs for communicating in sign language, ___% of the time.

*13. Draw ___ (number) vertical lines connecting two parallel lines which are ___ (number) inches apart, using only isolated finger movements, ___ out of ___ times.

*14. Draw ___ (number) circles between two parallel lines which are ___ (number) inches apart, using only isolated finger movements, ___ out of ___ times.

(continued)

* These objectives are skills to be observed within the classroom setting. They may be especially useful in the total team-generated IEP models.

Graphomotor
 a. manuscript
 b. cursive
 c. upper
 d. lower

NOTES

*15. Draw ___ *(number)* connected loops between two parallel lines which are ___ *(number)* inches apart, using only isolated finger movements, ___ out of ___ times.

*16. Use isolated finger movements to write the alphabet in ___ *(upper/lower)*-case ___ *(manuscript/cursive)* writing, for ___ *(number)* of the 26 letters.

Customized objectives:

* These objectives are skills to be observed within the classroom setting. They may be especially useful in the total team-generated IEP models.

Long-Term Goal 3

To improve functional shoulder, arm, and hand control for greater success with fine motor tasks and classroom and home manipulatives.

Objective I

To demonstrate in-hand manipulation, _____(child's name) will:

*1. Form a spaghetti-like strand of clay or dough by rolling the clay between the thumb and first two fingertips, ___ out of ___ times.

2. Form a ball from a ___-inch piece of paper with one hand, ___ out of ___ times.

3. Grasp and then place a ___-inch peg using only the same hand for any change in orientation, ___ out of ___ times.

4. Pick up ___ (number) small pegs, one at a time, and retain them in the palm of same hand, ___ out of ___ times.

5. Move a rubber band from around finger MCP joints (knuckles) to the fingertips and thumb, using thumb and finger movements only, ___ out of ___ times.

6. Move a rubber band from around index and middle finger MCP joints (knuckles) to fingertips and thumb, using thumb and finger movements only, ___ out of ___ times.

7. Hold and then move a coin or chip from palm of hand to fingertips, using same hand, ___ out of ___ times.

Objective I-5

*8. Hold and sort ___ (number) cards, one at a time, with one hand, ___ out of ___ times.

*9. Hold and sort ___ (number) coins, one at a time, with one hand, ___ out of ___ times.

*10. Alternately sort ___ (number) paper clips and ___ (number) pennies from the palm of the same hand, within ___ (number) attempts.

11. Hold ___ (number) pegs in palm of hand and, using same hand, place pegs one at a time into pegboard without dropping any, ___ out of ___ times.

12. Spin a small top or jack, ___ out of ___ times.

(continued)

* These objectives are skills to be observed within the classroom setting. They may be especially useful in the total team-generated IEP models.

*13. Twist an object (for example, a tube cap, knob, screw, or combination lock) using only thumb and finger movements, ___% of the time.

*14. Hold pencil in the air with tripod grasp and walk fingers up and down pencil shaft ___ *(number)* times, using ___ *(number)* steps.

*15. Hold pencil in air with tripod grasp and fully rotate so that markings on pencil shaft move in a clockwise direction, then counterclockwise, ___ *(number)* consecutive times each.

*16. Twirl pencil in a complete circular pattern, passing it end-over-end using only thumb, index, and middle fingers, ___ *(number)* consecutive times.

*17. Reposition pencil from writing position to erasing position, using only one hand, ___ out of ___ times.

Customized objectives:

* These objectives are skills to be observed within the classroom setting. They may be especially useful in the total team-generated IEP models.

Long-Term Goal 3

To improve functional shoulder, arm, and hand control for greater success with fine motor tasks and classroom and home manipulatives.

Objective J

To demonstrate prescissor skills, _____(child's name) will:

1. Use squeeze tongs to pick up and release ___ (number) cotton balls.

2. Use squeeze tongs to pick up and release ___ (number) one-inch blocks.

3. Use squeeze tongs to pick up and release ___ (number) marbles.

4. Use squeeze tongs to pick up and release ___ (number) small objects.

5. Use scissor tongs to pick up and release ___ (number) cotton balls.

6. Use scissor tongs to pick up and release ___ (number) one-inch blocks.

7. Use scissor tongs to pick up and release ___ (number) marbles.

8. Use scissor tongs to pick up and release ___ (number) small items.

9. Use tweezers to pick up and release ___ (number) small objects.

*10. Use a hole punch to punch ___ (number) holes on dots.

11. Use tongs to pick up and release items (for example, food from salad bar).

Customized objectives:

* These objectives are skills to be observed within the classroom setting. They may be especially useful in the total team-generated IEP models.

Long-Term Goal 3

To improve functional shoulder, arm, and hand control for greater success with fine motor tasks and classroom and home manipulatives.

Objective K

Objectives 1 through 13 are task oriented. Objectives 14 through 21 are quality oriented. Objectives from both areas are recommended.

To develop and refine scissor skills using appropriate hand positioning, _____(child's name) will:

Task-Oriented Objectives:

  *1. Use one hand to open and close ___ *(Classroom Tool)* ___ times consecutively.

  *2. Snip edge of paper ___ times, using ___ *(Classroom Tool)*.

  *3. Cut off pieces of paper, using ___ *(Classroom Tool)*.

  *4. Cut paper with ___ *(number)* consecutive movements, using ___ *(Classroom Tool)*.

  *5. Cut completely across a ___-inch paper, using ___ *(Classroom Tool)*.

  *6. Cut along a ___-inch line, within ___-inch accuracy, using ___ *(Classroom Tool)*.

  *7. Cut along a ___-inch zigzag line containing ___ *(number)* diagonals, within ___-inch accuracy, using ___ *(Classroom Tool)*.

  *8. Cut along a ___-inch S-curved line, with ___-inch accuracy, using ___ *(Classroom Tool)*.

  *9. Cut out a ___-inch square, with ___-inch accuracy, using ___ *(Classroom Tool)*.

  *10. Cut out a ___-inch triangle, with ___-inch accuracy, using ___ *(Classroom Tool)*.

  *11. Cut out a ___-inch circle, with ___-inch accuracy, using ___ *(Classroom Tool)*.

  *12. Cut out a simple ___-inch form containing angles and curves, with ___-inch accuracy, using ___ *(Classroom Tool)*.

  *13. Cut out a complex ___-inch form containing angles and curves, with ___-inch accuracy, using ___ *(Classroom Tool)*.

(continued)

* These objectives are skills to be observed within the classroom setting. They may be especially useful in the total team-generated IEP models.

Classroom Tools
a. standard classroom scissors
b. squeeze or easy-grip scissors
c. adapted scissors
d. sharp scissors
e. ruler
f. stapler
g. compass
h. hole punch
i. pencil sharpener
j. one-inch blade scissors
k. tape dispenser

NOTES

Long-Term Goal 3, Objective K (continued)

Quality-Oriented Objectives:

*14. Cut using a neutral (thumbs up) approach with both hands, ___% of the time, using ___ *(Classroom Tool)*.

*15. Reposition the paper-holding hand while cutting, ___% of the time.

*16. Attend to details such as sharp corners or rounded edges when cutting, ___% of the time.

*17. Cut, using a balance of thumb and finger flexion and extension, ___% of the time, using ___ *(Classroom Tool)*.

*18. Cut, grasping the scissors with the thumb and first two fingers, ___% of the time, using ___ *(Classroom Tool)*.

*19. Cut, grasping the scissors with the thumb and middle or index finger, ___% of the time, using ___ *(Classroom Tool)*.

*20. Cut paper, opening and closing scissor blades only halfway, ___% of the time.

*21. Cut, with scissor holes maintained at the middle of the thumb and fingers, ___% of the time.

Customized objectives:

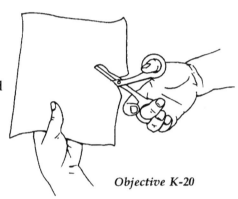

Objective K-20

* These objectives are skills to be observed within the classroom setting. They may be especially useful in the total team-generated IEP models.

QUALIFIERS

Hand/Foot Usage
  c. bilateral
  e. right
  f. left

Body Parts
  i. index finger
  j. long/middle finger
  k. ring finger
  l. little (pinky) finger

Body Movements
  a. flexion
  b. extension
  c. abduction
  d. adduction
  e. external rotation
  f. internal rotation
  g. ulnar deviation
  h. radial deviation
  i. pronation/pronated
  j. supination/supinated
  k. opposition/opposed
  l. neutral
  m. (any combination of above)

NOTES

Long-Term Goal 3

To improve functional shoulder, arm, and hand control for greater success with fine motor tasks and classroom and home manipulatives.

Objective L

To maintain or improve passive range of motion, needed for activities such as reaching and self-help tasks, _____(*child's name*) will:

1. Allow/tolerate ___ (*number*) degrees of ___ (*Hand/Foot Usage*) shoulder ___ (*Body Movement*).

2. Allow/tolerate ___ (*number*) degrees of ___ (*Hand/Foot Usage*) elbow ___ (*Body Movement*).

3. Allow/tolerate ___ (*number*) degrees of ___ (*Hand/Foot Usage*) forearm ___ (*Body Movement*).

4. Allow/tolerate ___ (*number*) degrees of ___ (*Hand/Foot Usage*) wrist ___ (*Body Movement*).

5. Allow/tolerate ___ (*number*) degrees of ___ (*Hand/Foot Usage*) thumb ___ (*Body Movement*).

6. Allow/tolerate ___ (*number*) degrees of ___ (*Hand/Foot Usage*) ___ (*Body Part*) finger ___ (*Body Movement*).

Customized objectives:

QUALIFIERS

Hand/Foot Usage
c. bilateral
e. right
f. left

Body Parts
i. index finger
j. long/middle finger
k. ring finger
l. little (pinky) finger

Body Movements
a. flexion
b. extension
c. abduction
d. adduction
e. external rotation
f. internal rotation
g. ulnar deviation
h. radial deviation
i. pronation/pronated
j. supination/supinated
k. opposition/opposed
l. neutral
m. (any combination of above)

NOTES

Long-Term Goal 3

To improve functional shoulder, arm, and hand control for greater success with fine motor tasks and classroom and home manipulatives.

Objective M

To maintain or improve active range of motion, needed for activities such as reaching and self-help tasks, _____(child's name) will:

1. Demonstrate ___ (number) degrees of ___ (Hand/Foot Usage) shoulder ___ (Body Movement).

2. Demonstrate ___ (number) degrees of ___ (Hand/Foot Usage) elbow ___ (Body Movement).

3. Demonstrate ___ (number) degrees of ___ (Hand/Foot Usage) forearm ___ (Body Movement).

4. Demonstrate ___ (number) degrees of ___ (Hand/Foot Usage) wrist ___ (Body Movement).

5. Demonstrate ___ (number) degrees of ___ (Hand/Foot Usage) thumb ___ (Body Movement).

6. Demonstrate ___ (number) degrees of ___ (Hand/Foot Usage) ___ (Body Part) finger ___ (Body Movement).

Customized objectives:

Long-Term Goal 3

To improve functional shoulder, arm, and hand control for greater success with fine motor tasks and classroom and home manipulatives.

Objective N

To maintain or improve functional range of motion, _____(*child's name*) will:

1. Extend involved arm(s) over head as in raising hand to answer a question.

2. Extend involved arm(s) out to the front (for example, reach for a pencil at top of desk).

3. Extend involved arm(s) to the sides (for example, to space self arm's distance apart for group activity).

4. Place hand(s) across chest, to touch opposite shoulder(s) (for example, to adjust coat).

5. Touch hand(s) to shoulder(s) on the same side.

6. Place hands behind the neck with elbows out to the side (for example, to adjust collar).

7. Put hands behind the back with the elbows out to the side, at waist level (for example, to tuck shirt into pants).

8. Turn palms up and down while keeping elbows flexed at sides (for example, to turn paper over and back).

9. Place palms together and raise elbows until forearms are horizontal across chest, for wrist extension (as if a seal clapping).

10. Move hand side to side, up and down at wrist, in a waving motion.

11. Make a tightly closed fist (for example, to crumple paper).

12. Open hand completely and spread fingers (for example, to trace hand).

Customized objectives:

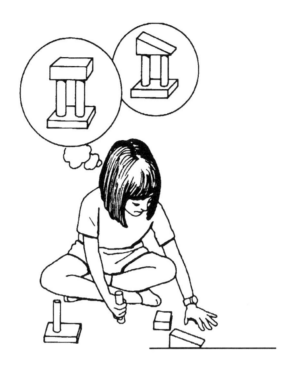

LONG-TERM GOAL
4

To improve motor planning to enhance quality of movement and efficient organization of self for effective participation in school and home activities.

Plane
a. horizontal
b. vertical
c. diagonal
d. circular
e. rotary
f. pendular
g. linear
h. forward
i. backward
j. sideways
k. forward, backward, and sideways
l. multidirectional

Graphomotor
a. manuscript
b. cursive
c. upper
d. lower
e. A to Z

Shapes
a. vertical line
b. horizontal line
c. circle
d. crossed lines
e. X
f. square
g. triangle
h. vertical diamond
i. horizontal diamond

NOTES

Long-Term Goal 4

To improve motor planning to enhance quality of movement and efficient organization of self for effective participation in school and home activities.

Objective A

To demonstrate improved awareness of positions and movements of body parts (proprioception/kinesthesia), _____(child's name) will:

1. With eyes closed, accurately duplicate an imposed position on self (as placed by therapist) on the opposite side of the body, executing ___ (number) positions.

2. With eyes closed, duplicate an imposed movement and accurately execute the same movement on the opposite side of body, performing ___ (number) movements.

*3. Trace a single ___-inch line ___ times and then, with eyes closed, draw the same length line, within ___-inch accuracy.

*4. Draw ___ (Plane) line on a chalkboard with eyes closed, correctly imitating the previously demonstrated visual and physical movement, ___ out of ___ times.

*5. Draw a ___ (Plane) line on paper with eyes closed, correctly imitating the previously demonstrated visual and physical movement, ___ out of ___ times.

*6. Form ___ (upper/lower)-case letter ___ (A to Z), using ___ (manuscript/ cursive) writing on the chalkboard, with eyes closed, correctly imitating the previously demonstrated visual and physical movement, ___ out of ___ times.

*7. Form ___ (upper/lower)-case letter ___ (A to Z), using ___ (manuscript/ cursive) writing on paper, with eyes closed, correctly imitating the previously demonstrated visual and physical movement, ___ out of ___ times.

*8. Write own name on paper, using ___ (manuscript/cursive) writing, with eyes closed, correctly imitating the previously demonstrated visual and physical movement, ___ out of ___ times.

*9. Imitate a ___ (Shape) recognizably, ___ out of ___ times.

*10. Grade pressure applied when writing or coloring so as not to break the implement or wrinkle or rip the paper, ___% of the time.

(continued)

* These objectives are skills to be observed within the classroom setting. They may be especially useful in the total team-generated IEP models.

QUALIFIERS
Graphomotor
a. manuscript
b. cursive
c. upper
d. lower
e. A to Z
NOTES

*11. Draw ___ *(number)* vertical lines connecting two parallel lines which are ___ inches apart, within ___-inch accuracy.

*12. Draw ___ *(number)* vertical lines connecting parallel lines ___ inches apart, using a top-to-bottom orientation, ___ out of ___ times.

*13. Copy ___ *(upper/lower)*-case letter(s)___ *(A to Z)*, in ___ *(manuscript, cursive)* writing, using correct directionality of letter formation, ___ out of ___ times.

*14. Copy the letters ___ *(A to Z)*, with proper formation, orientation, and closure, ___ out of ___ times.

*15. Form *(upper/lower)*-case letter(s) ___ *(A to Z)*, on request, in ___ *(manuscript/cursive)* writing, using correct directionality of letter formation, ___ out of ___ times.

Customized objectives:

* These objectives are skills to be observed within the classroom setting. They may be especially useful in the total team-generated IEP models.

Long-Term Goal 4

To improve motor planning to enhance quality of movement and efficient organization of self for effective participation in school and home activities.

Objective B

To demonstrate the ability to generate (think of) ideas for action, _____(*child's name*) will:

*1. Physically or verbally communicate ___ *(number)* ideas for play or work activities without cues.

*2. Physically or verbally communicate ___ *(number)* ideas for play or work activities with ___ *(number)* cues by therapist.

*3. Physically or verbally communicate ___ *(number)* ideas for play or work activities when presented with ___ *(number)* choices.

Customized objectives:

* These objectives are skills to be observed within the classroom setting. They may be especially useful in the total team-generated IEP models.

Long-Term Goal 4

To improve motor planning to enhance quality of movement and efficient organization of self for effective participation in school and home activities.

Objective C

To demonstrate the improved ability to plan a course of action,_____ (*child's name*) will:

*1. Specify at least ___ *(number)* steps needed to correctly sequence the movements required to perform a given task.

*2. Communicate ___ *(number)* ideas of how to motorically interact with ___ *(specify object)*.

*3. Specify how to accomplish ___ *(number)* components of an obstacle course consisting of ___ *(specify objects)*.

Customized objectives:

* These objectives are skills to be observed within the classroom setting. They may be especially useful in the total team-generated IEP models.

Long-Term Goal 4

To improve motor planning to enhance quality of movement and efficient organization of self for effective participation in school and home activities.

Objective D

To demonstrate the improved ability to execute movement(s),_____ (*child's name*) will:

1. Assume ___ *(number)* postures that involve movement of only one arm or leg, within ___ *(number)* seconds of demonstration.

2. Assume ___ *(number)* symmetrical postures, within ___ *(number)* seconds of each demonstration (for example, raise both hands above head at the same time).

3. Assume ___ *(number)* asymmetrical postures involving ___ *(number)* body parts, within ___ *(number)* seconds of each demonstration (for example, simultaneously cross ankles, touch head and hip).

*4. Perform ___ *(number)* continuous movements of only one arm or leg, within ___ *(number)* seconds of demonstration and sustain the movements for ___ *(number)* seconds (for example, turn handle of pencil sharpener, diadokokinesis).

*5. Perform ___ *(number)* continuous symmetrical movements, within ___ *(number)* seconds of the demonstration and sustain the movement for ___ *(number)* seconds (for example, jumping, clapping, doing jumping jacks).

*6. Catch a bounced ___-inch ball outside of arm's reach, requiring a postural adjustment, ___ out of ___ times.

7. Perform ___ *(number)* continuous asymmetrical movements involving ___ *(number)* body parts, within ___ *(number)* seconds of demonstration and sustain for ___ *(number)* seconds (for example, hopping, bilateral finger-nose test).

8. Perform ___ *(number)* simultaneous reciprocal movements involving ___ *(number)* body parts, within ___ *(number)* seconds of demonstration, and sustain for ___ *(number)* seconds (for example, skipping, alternating fists).

*9. Join both sides of jacket zipper and zip coat, within ___ *(number)* attempts.

*10. Independently open milk carton without spilling.

(continued)

Objective D-8

* These objectives are skills to be observed within the classroom setting. They may be especially useful in the total team-generated IEP models.

Long-Term Goal 4, Objective D (continued)

*11. Independently open milk carton without spilling, within ___ *(number)* seconds.

*12. Independently place a rubber band around a variety of objects to keep them closed or bound, ___ out of ___ times.

13. Independently pump a swing after an initial push, sustaining the swing's motion for ___ minutes.

14. Independently move a swing using a pumping action from a stopped position, sustaining the swing's motion for ___ minutes.

15. Jump rope ___ consecutive times.

*16. Execute a ___ *(number)*-step ___ *(Hand/Foot Usage)* task, given only verbal direction, within ___ *(number)* seconds.

*17. Complete a specific ___ *(number)*-step activity as demonstrated (for example, packing a book bag, completing an obstacle course, folding a paper airplane).

*18. Complete a specific ___ *(number)*-step activity following verbal directions (for example, packing a book bag, completing an obstacle course, folding a paper airplane).

*19. Complete a specific ___ *(number)*-step activity with only initial directions (for example, packing a book bag, completing an obstacle course, folding a paper airplane).

*20. Complete a specific ___ *(number)*-step activity without direction (for example, packing a book bag, completing an obstacle course, folding a paper airplane).

*21. Follow a ___ *(number)*-step direction with ___ *(Degree of Assistance)* ___ *(Type of Assistance)*, ___% of the time.

Customized objectives:

---

* These objectives are skills to be observed within the classroom setting. They may be especially useful in the total team-generated IEP models.

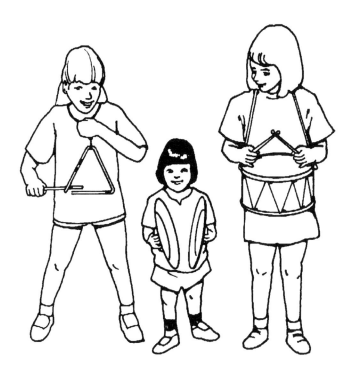

LONG-TERM GOAL
5

To improve bilateral coordination to enhance movement efficiency and functional participation in school and home activities.

Long-Term Goal 5

To improve bilateral coordination to enhance movement efficiency and functional participation in school and home activities.

Objective A

To demonstrate efficient crossing midline of the body, _____(child's name) will:

*1. Use one hand to retrieve and/or place ___ (number) objects on the opposite side of the body.

2. Trace over a ___-inch horizontal figure-8 pattern ___ times, while sitting at a desk, with minimal displacement or turning of body from midline no more than ___ time(s).

3. Trace over a ___-inch horizontal figure-8 pattern ___ times, while standing, with minimal displacement or turning of body from the midline no more than ___ time(s).

4. Complete ___ (number) consecutive crossover patterns of a clapping hand song (for example, patty cake), within ___ (number) seconds.

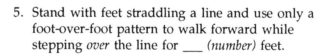
Objective A-5

5. Stand with feet straddling a line and use only a foot-over-foot pattern to walk forward while stepping *over* the line for ___ (number) feet.

6. Use only a foot-over-foot pattern to walk sideways along a ___-foot long line and return while facing in the same direction.

7. Spontaneously cross midline when appropriate to the task, ___% of the time.

Customized objectives:

Objective A-6

* These objectives are skills to be observed within the classroom setting. They may be especially useful in the total team-generated IEP models.

Long-Term Goal 5

To improve bilateral coordination to enhance movement efficiency and functional participation in school and home activities.

Objective B

To demonstrate the ability to simultaneously use both sides of the body to perform the same movements (symmetrical), _____(child's name) will:

1. Push a rolling ___ (Type of Ball) ball to wall or partner ___ (number) consecutive times.

*2. Throw a ___-inch ball from midline of body to within 20 degrees of partner, or target, ___ out of ___ times.

*3. Catch a ___-inch ball with hands, ___ out of ___ times.

4. Jump up and land with both feet together, ___ (number) consecutive times.

5. Jump forward with both feet together, ___ (number) consecutive times, within ___ (number) seconds.

*6. Pull apart ___ (number) ___ (Size) pop-beads.

*7. Push together ___ (number) ___ (Size) pop-beads.

*8. Scoop up a quantity of small objects or sand with the hands, and transfer into a container which is ___ inches away, without separating hands until reaching the container.

9. Remove ___ (number) pairs of ___-inch pegs from a pegboard, with both hands, and place into a container at midline.

10. Propel self forward, using hands symmetrically ___ (number) times while prone on a scooterboard, ___ out of ___ times.

11. Propel self forward, using feet symmetrically, ___ (number) times, while sitting on a scooterboard, ___ out of ___ times.

12. Drop a ___-inch ball from midline and, after one bounce, catch it with both hands, ___ out of ___ times.

13. Hit a ___ (Type of Ball) ball against a wall ___ (number) consecutive times, using hands symmetrically.

14. Kick a rolled ___ (Type of Ball) ball with both feet ___ (number) consecutive times while sitting on floor and leaning back on extended arms.

(continued)

* These objectives are skills to be observed within the classroom setting. They may be especially useful in the total team-generated IEP models.

QUALIFIERS

Plane
a. horizontal
b. vertical
c. diagonal
d. circular
e. rotary
f. pendular
g. linear
h. forward
i. backward
j. sideways
k. forward, backward, and sideways
l. multidirectional

NOTES

*15. Carry lunch tray with both hands successfully.

16. Simultaneously draw ___ (number) pairs of ___ (Plane) lines on chalkboard, using both hands.

17. Simultaneously draw ___ (number) pairs of ___ (Plane) lines on paper, using both hands.

18. Move two streamers away from the body, using arms in a circular pattern starting at midline, ___ (number) consecutive times.

19. Perform ___ (number) jumping jacks, within ___ (number) seconds.

Customized objectives:

* These objectives are skills to be observed within the classroom setting. They may be especially useful in the total team-generated IEP models.

Sizes
 a. small
 b. medium
 c. large
 d. ___-inch

Degree of Assistance
 a. minimum(ly)
 b. moderate(ly)
 c. maximum(ly)
 d. verbal
 e. hand-over-hand
 f. physical
 g. tactile
 h. auditory
 i. visual
 j. no
 k. (any combination of above)

Type of Assistance
 a. assistance
 b. supervision
 c. guidance
 d. prompt
 e. demonstration
 f. cues
 g. in functional activities
 h. independently
 i. with gravity (assisted)
 j. gravity eliminated
 k. against gravity
 l. with ___ facilitation to ___
 m. with adapted devices
 n. passive
 o. active
 p. adaptive techniques
 q. (any combination of above)

NOTES

Long-Term Goal 5

To improve bilateral coordination to enhance movement efficiency and functional participation in school and home activities.

Objective C

To demonstrate the ability to simultaneously use both hands/sides of the body to perform different movements (asymmetrical), _____(child's name) will:

1. Use involved extremity as a functional assist, ___% of the time.

*2. Consistently stabilize a bowl with one hand while stirring or scooping food with a spoon held in the other hand.

*3. Successfully open a ___-inch jar, using one hand to stabilize the jar and the other to unscrew the lid, ___ out of ___ times.

*4. Open door with one arm while holding objects in other arm, ___ out of ___ times.

*5. Stabilize paper with one hand while coloring or writing with the other, ___% of the time.

6. String ___ (number) ___-inch beads, using one hand to pick up and manipulate the bead and the other hand to manage the string.

7. Successfully unscrew a nut from a ___-inch bolt or screw, ___ out of ___ times.

*8. Open a 1/2-pint milk carton, using both hands, ___ out of ___ times.

*9. Accurately pour liquid from a 1/2-pint container into a small drinking cup held in the other hand, ___% of the time.

*10. Successfully sharpen a pencil, using a manual classroom pencil sharpener, ___% of the time.

*11. Hold ruler in place with one hand (nondominant) while drawing a straight line along the ruler edge with the other hand (dominant), ___ out of ___ times.

*12. Completely erase pencil markings without wrinkling or ripping the paper, ___% of the time.

*13. Hold a stencil in place while drawing along the stencil edges, with fewer than ___ (number) slips.

*14. Tie shoelaces in a bow with ___ (Degree of Assistance) ___ (Type of Assistance), ___% of the time.

Customized objectives:

* These objectives are skills to be observed within the classroom setting. They may be especially useful in the total team-generated IEP models.

Type of Ball
  a. volley
  b. beach
  c. ___-inch playground
  d. ___-inch therapy
  e. hard
  f. tennis
  g. basket
  h. ___-inch foam
  i. base
  j. medicine
  k. racket
  l. Wiffle®
  m. cage

NOTES

Wiffle® is a registered trademark of The Wiffle Ball, Inc., Shelton, CT.

Long-Term Goal 5

To improve bilateral coordination to enhance movement efficiency and functional participation in school and home activities.

Objective D

To demonstrate ability to simultaneously use both sides of the body to perform rhythmical reciprocal movements, _____(*child's name*) will:

1. Crawl on hands and knees for a distance of ___ (*number*) feet.

2. Propel self forward, using feet in a walking pattern, for a distance of ___ (*number*) feet, while sitting on a scooterboard.

3. Propel self forward, using hands alternately, for a distance of ___ (*number*) feet, while prone on a scooterboard.

*4. Ascend ___ (*number*) steps, placing only one foot on each step. (Hand support permitted.)

*5. Descend ___ (*number*) steps, placing only one foot on each step. (Hand support permitted.)

6. Use a foot-driven stationary or mobile car or bike, for ___ (*number*) minutes.

7. Use a hand-driven stationary or mobile car or bike, for ___ (*number*) minutes.

8. Pull ___ (*number*) feet of rope to self, using a hand-over-hand pattern, while sitting.

9. Wring or twist a washcloth ___ times.

10. Hit a balloon into the air, using hands in alternating pattern, ___ (*number*) consecutive times.

11. Bounce a ___ (*Type of Ball*) ball, using hands in alternating pattern, ___ (*number*) consecutive times.

12. Open the fingers of one fisted hand while forming a fist with the other hand, ___ times, alternating fists.

13. Alternately tap isolated index fingers while wrists are stabilized, for ___ (*number*) sets.

Customized objectives:

* These objectives are skills to be observed within the classroom setting. They may be especially useful in the total team-generated IEP models.

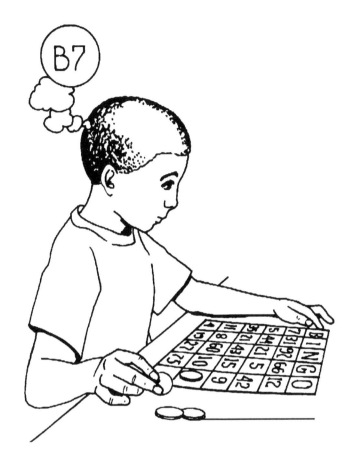

LONG-TERM GOAL
6

To improve ocular motor control for greater success in reading, writing, copying, and eye-hand coordination tasks.

Duration
- a. seconds
- b. minutes
- c. repetitions

Degree of Assistance
- a. minimum(ly)
- b. moderate(ly)
- c. maximum(ly)
- d. verbal
- e. hand-over-hand
- f. physical
- g. tactile
- h. auditory
- i. visual
- j. no
- k. (any combination of above)

Type of Assistance
- a. assistance
- b. supervision
- c. guidance
- d. prompt
- e. demonstration
- f. cues
- g. in functional activities
- h. independently
- i. with gravity (assisted)
- j. gravity eliminated
- k. against gravity
- l. with ___ facilitation to ___
- m. with adapted devices
- n. passive
- o. active
- p. adaptive techniques
- q. (any combination of above)

NOTES

Long-Term Goal 6

To improve ocular motor control for greater success in reading, writing, copying, and eye-hand coordination tasks.

Objective A

To demonstrate visual focusing skills, _____ (*child's name*) will:

*1. Focus for ___ seconds on the face of the person speaking.

*2. Focus for ___ seconds on an object being held or manipulated.

*3. Maintain visual focus on task for ___ *(number)* ___ *(Duration)* with ___ *(Degree of Assistance)* ___ *(Type of Assistance)* ___% of the time.

Customized objectives:

---

* These objectives are skills to be observed within the classroom setting. They may be especially useful in the total team-generated IEP models.

Plane
a. horizontal
b. vertical
c. diagonal
d. circular
e. rotary
f. pendular
g. linear
h. forward
i. backward
j. sideways
k. forward, backward, and sideways
l. multidirectional

NOTES

Long-Term Goal 6

To improve ocular motor control for greater success in reading, writing, copying, and eye-hand coordination tasks.

Objective B

To demonstrate visual tracking, _____(child's name) will:

1. Maintain visual contact with a descending balloon from ___ (number) feet above head to the floor.

2. Successfully follow a Wiffle® ball suspended from a ___ (number)-foot string as it swings horizontally at eye level, for ___ (number) seconds.

3. Follow a brightly colored object placed 12 inches from face in a ___ (Plane) plane, using binocular coordination, ___ out of ___ times.

4. Maintain visual contact for ___ (number) seconds with a car or marble as it races through a multiplane track.

*5. Disassociate eye movements from the head during functional activities, ___% of the time.

6. Use disassociated eye movements from the head to successfully follow a Wiffle® ball suspended from a ___ (number)-foot string as it swings horizontally at eye level, for ___ (number) seconds.

7. Use disassociated eye from head movements to maintain visual contact with a variable speed and direction wind-up toy, for ___ (number) seconds.

8. Use disassociated eye movements from the head to maintain visual contact with a car or marble as it races through a multiplane track, for ___ (number) seconds.

*9. Maintain visual contact while the teacher is moving about the room, ___% of the time.

*10. Follow the second hand of a classroom clock for ___ (number) seconds and correctly indicate as it passes over each number, successfully tracking for ___ (number) seconds.

11. Maintain visual contact with a variable speed and direction wind-up toy, for ___ (number) seconds.

Customized objectives:

___
Wiffle® is a registered trademark of The Wiffle Ball, Inc., Shelton, CT.

* These objectives are skills to be observed within the classroom setting. They may be especially useful in the total team-generated IEP models.

QUALIFIERS

Shape
  a. vertical line
  b. horizontal line
  c. circle
  d. crossed lines
  e. X
  f. square
  g. triangle
  h. vertical diamond
  i. horizontal diamond

Graphomotor
  e. A to Z

NOTES

Long-Term Goal 6

To improve ocular motor control for greater success in reading, writing, copying, and eye-hand coordination tasks.

Objective C

To demonstrate visual scanning abilities, _____(child's name) will:

*1. Locate a named object from a shelf or closet, within ___ (number) seconds.

*2. Locate ___ (number) indicated pictures or numbers on a bingo card, within ___ (number) seconds.

*3. Locate the letters ___ (A to Z) from ___ (number) standard typed lines, with ___% accuracy, in ___ (number) seconds.

*4. Locate the number(s) ___ from ___ (number) vertical columns comprised of 10 numbers each, spaced ___ inches apart, with ___% accuracy, in ___ (number) seconds.

*5. Locate alphabet keys on keyboard by typing alphabet, within ___ (number) seconds.

*6. Draw a straight line within a ___-inch wide path without touching sides for a distance of ___ inches.

*7. Draw a line within a ___-inch wide 5-inch long horizontal S-curved path without touching the sides.

*8. Trace along a ___-inch ___ (Shape) with ___-inch accuracy.

*9. Trace along a ___-inch zigzag line consisting of ___ (number) diagonals, with ___-inch accuracy.

Customized objectives:

---

* These objectives are skills to be observed within the classroom setting. They may be especially useful in the total team-generated IEP models.

Long-Term Goal 6

To improve ocular motor control for greater success in reading, writing, copying, and eye-hand coordination tasks.

Objective D

To demonstrate functional visual localization, _____(child's name) will:

*1. Connect ___ (number) dots which are ___ inches apart, using straight lines, within ___-inch accuracy from the side of the dots.

*2. Sequentially connect a picture or design composed of ___ (number) dots, within ___-inch accuracy, in ___ (number) seconds.

*3. Connect a picture or design composed of ___ (number) dots, within ___-inch accuracy, in ___ (number) seconds.

*4. Copy ___ (number) letters or numbers from a paper, with ___% accuracy, in ___ (number) seconds.

*5. Copy ___ (number) letters or numbers from the chalkboard, with ___% accuracy, in ___ (number) seconds.

*6. Copy a sentence which is composed of ___ (number) words from a paper or book, with ___% accuracy, in ___ (number) seconds.

*7. Copy a sentence which is composed of ___ (number) words from the chalkboard, with ___% accuracy, in ___ (number) seconds.

Customized objectives:

* These objectives are skills to be observed within the classroom setting. They may be especially useful in the total team-generated IEP models.

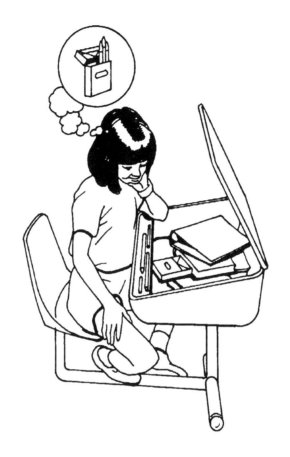

LONG-TERM GOAL
7

To improve visual perception and/or perceptual motor skills for greater success in academics and written work.

Long-Term Goal 7

To improve visual perception and/or perceptual motor skills for greater success in academics and written work.

Objective A

To demonstrate improved body awareness, _____(child's name) will:

*1. Point to ___ (number) specified body parts on self.

*2. Point to ___ (number) specified body parts on others.

*3. Point to ___ (number) specified body parts on a doll.

*4. Point to ___ (number) specified body parts on self and others.

*5. Name ___ (number) body parts on self.

*6. Name ___ (number) body parts on others.

*7. Name ___ (number) body parts on a doll.

*8. Name ___ (number) body parts on self and others.

*9. Point to ___ (number) specified joints on self.

*10. Point to ___ (number) specified joints on others.

*11. Point to ___ (number) specified joints on self and others.

*12. Name ___ (number) specified joints on self.

*13. Name ___ (number) specified joints on others.

*14. Name ___ (number) specified joints on self and others.

*15. Indicate right/left side of body on self.

*16. Indicate right/left side of body on others.

*17. Indicate right/left side of body on self and others.

*18. Indicate ___ (number) body parts, including right- or left-sidedness on self, within ___ (number) seconds.

*19. Indicate ___ (number) body parts, including right- or left-sidedness on others, within ___ (number) seconds.

(continued)

* These objectives are skills to be observed within the classroom setting. They may be especially useful in the total team-generated IEP models.

Long-Term Goal 7, Objective A (continued)

*20. Indicate ___ *(number)* body parts, including right- or left-sidedness on self and others, within ___ *(number)* seconds.

*21. With ___ *(Degree of Assistance)* ___ *(Type of Assistance)*, touch one body part to another on self upon request, within ___ *(number)* seconds. (For example, "Put your elbow on your knee.")

*22. Draw a person, with ___ *(number)* body parts.

*23. With ___ *(Degree of Assistance)* ___ *(Type of Assistance)*, name the specified body part and the side of another person when asked, "What is this?" ___% of the time.

Customized objectives:

---

* These objectives are skills to be observed within the classroom setting. They may be especially useful in the total team-generated IEP models.

QUALIFIERS

Plane
a. horizontal
b. vertical
c. diagonal
d. circular
e. rotary
f. pendular
g. linear
h. forward
i. backward
j. sideways
k. forward, backward, and sideways
l. multidirectional

Degree of Assistance
a. minimum(ly)
b. moderate(ly)
c. maximum(ly)
d. verbal
e. hand-over-hand
f. physical
g. tactile
h. auditory
i. visual
j. no
k. (any combination of above)

Type of Assistance
a. assistance
b. supervision
c. guidance
d. prompt
e. demonstration
f. cues
g. in functional activities
h. independently
i. with gravity (assisted)
j. gravity eliminated
k. against gravity
l. with ___ facilitation to ___
m. with adapted devices
n. passive
o. active
p. adaptive techniques
q. (any combination of above)

Spatial Concepts
a. in/out of
b. on/off of
c. under/over
d. in front of/ in back of
e. next to/beside
f. through
g. up/down
h. behind

Long-Term Goal 7

To improve visual perception and/or perceptual motor skills for greater success in academics and written work.

Objective B

To demonstrate improved spatial awareness of self in space and the relationship of self to objects and the environment, _____(child's name) will:

*1. Move in ___ (Plane) direction when verbally cued, ___ out of ___ times, within ___ (number) seconds.

*2. With — (Degree of Assistance) ___ (Type of Assistance), move self ___ (Spatial Concept) an object, ___% of the time.

*3. With ___ (Degree of Assistance) ___ (Type of Assistance), move body part in (Plane h, i, j, k) direction, ___% of the time.

*4. With ___ (Degree of Assistance) ___ (Type of Assistance), place an object ___ (Spatial Concept c, d, e) self, ___% of the time.

*5. With ___ (Degree of Assistance) ___ (Type of Assistance), assemble a ___ (number)-piece body part puzzle within its frame, ___% of the time.

*6. With ___ (Degree of Assistance) ___ (Type of Assistance), assemble a ___ (number)-piece body part puzzle without a frame, ___% of the time.

*7. With ___ (Degree of Assistance) ___ (Type of Assistance), describe the orientation of one body part to another, ___% of the time. (For example, eyes are above mouth.)

*8. ___% of the time, identify right/left side of body being touched, within ___ (number) seconds.

*9. With ___ (Degree of Assistance) ___ (Type of Assistance), touch right or left side of person with back to self, ___% of the time.

*10. Upon request, with ___ (Degree of Assistance) ___ (Type of Assistance), touch right or left side of person facing self, ___% of the time.

*11. With ___ (Degree of Assistance) ___ (Type of Assistance), name the specified body part and the side of another person when asked "What is this?" ___% of the time.

(continued)

---

* These objectives are skills to be observed within the classroom setting. They may be especially useful in the total team-generated IEP models.

QUALIFIERS

Plane
  a. horizontal
  b. vertical
  c. diagonal
  d. circular
  e. rotary
  f. pendular
  g. linear
  h. forward
  i. backward
  j. sideways
  k. forward, backward, and sideways
  l. multidirectional

Degree of Assistance
  a. minimum(ly)
  b. moderate(ly)
  c. maximum(ly)
  d. verbal
  e. hand-over-hand
  f. physical
  g. tactile
  h. auditory
  i. visual
  j. no
  k. (any combination of above)

Type of Assistance
  a. assistance
  b. supervision
  c. guidance
  d. prompt
  e. demonstration
  f. cues
  g. in functional activities
  h. independently
  i. with gravity (assisted)
  j. gravity eliminated
  k. against gravity
  l. with ___ facilitation to ___
  m. with adapted devices
  n. passive
  o. active
  p. adaptive techniques
  q. (any combination of above)

Dressing
  a. coats/sweaters
  b. hat
  c. gloves/mittens
  d. boots
  e. shoes
  f. socks
  g. button-down smock/ shirt
  h. pullover smock/shirt
  i. belt
  j. braces/orthotics
  k. clothes

Long-Term Goal 7, Objective B (continued)

*12. Put on ___ *(Dressing)* in the appropriate orientation with ___ *(Degree of Assistance)* ___ *(Type of Assistance)*, ___% of the time.

*13. Demonstrate the ability to navigate to familiar places within the environment, with ___ *(Degree of Assistance)* ___ *(Type of Assistance)*, ___% of the time.

*14. Maneuver through the environment while maintaining the condition of self, materials, and surroundings, with ___ *(Degree of Assistance)* ___ *(Type of Assistance)*, ___% of the time.

*15. Move in ___ *(Plane)* direction when verbally cued, ___ out of ___ times, within ___ *(number)* seconds.

*16. Form horizontal line on paper, moving from left to right, ___ out of ___ times, with verbal cues only.

*17. Form left-to-right and right-to-left diagonal lines on paper, ___ out of ___ times, with verbal cues only.

Customized objectives:

---

* These objectives are skills to be observed within the classroom setting. They may be especially useful in the total team-generated IEP models.

Long-Term Goal 7

To improve visual perception and/or perceptual motor skills for greater success in academics and written work.

Objective C

To demonstrate improved awareness of forms and spatial relations of objects to each other, _____(*child's name*) will:

*1. Place ___ (*number*) scattered forms into a ___ (*number*)-piece formboard, with ___ (*number*) attempt(s) per piece.

*2. Complete ___ (*number*)-piece noninterlocking puzzles.

*3. Complete ___ (*number*)-piece interlocking puzzles within a frame.

*4. Complete ___ (*number*)-piece interlocking puzzles without a frame.

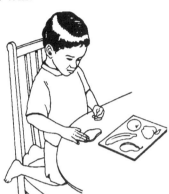

Objective C-2

5. Imitate a 3- or 4-cube train, within ___ (*number*) attempts.

6. Copy a 3- or 4-cube train, within ___ (*number*) attempts.

7. Imitate a 3-cube bridge, within ___ (*number*) attempts.

8. Copy a 3-cube bridge, within ___ (*number*) attempts.

9. Imitate a 5-cube gate, within ___ (*number*) attempts.

10. Copy a 5-cube gate, within ___ (*number*) attempts.

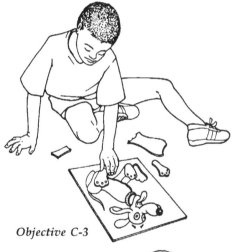

Objective C-3

11. Imitate a 6-cube step design, within ___ (*number*) attempts.

12. Copy a 6-cube step design, within ___ (*number*) attempts.

13. Imitate a 6-cube pyramid design, within ___ (*number*) attempts.

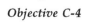

Objective C-4

(continued)

* These objectives are skills to be observed within the classroom setting. They may be especially useful in the total team-generated IEP models.

QUALIFIERS

Spatial Concepts
a. in/out of
b. on/off of
c. under/over
d. in front of/
   in back of
e. next to/beside
f. through
g. up/down
h. behind

School-Related Activities
a. physical education
b. playground
c. classroom
d. fine motor
e. gross motor
f. postural
g. desk top
h. (any specific activity
   of your choice)

NOTES

Long-Term Goal 7, Objective C (continued)

14. Copy a 6-cube pyramid design, within ___ *(number)* attempts.

15. Imitate a 10-cube step design, within ___ *(number)* attempts.

16. Copy a 10-cube step design, within ___ *(number)* attempts.

17. Imitate a ___ *(number)*-cube design, within ___ *(number)* attempts.

18. Copy a ___ *(number)*-cube design, within ___ *(number)* attempts.

19. Imitate age-appropriate cube designs, within ___ *(number)* attempts.

20. Copy age-appropriate cube designs, within ___ *(number)* attempts.

21. Construct a ___ *(number)*-cube design from a picture, within ___ *(number)* attempts.

22. Correctly orient an object/picture when it is displaced in space, within ___ *(number)* attempts.

*23. Indicate which stimulus is in a different spatial orientation from the other ___ *(number)* presented, ___ out of ___ times.

*24. Place an object ___ *(Spatial Concept)* another object, upon verbal command, within ___ *(number)* attempts.

*25. Join a picture divided into ___ *(number)* pieces, within ___ *(number)* attempts.

*26. Join a shape divided into ___ *(number)* pieces, within ___ *(number)* attempts.

*27. Identify the right or left side of the paper, ___% of the time.

*28. Draw ___ *(number)* vertical lines connecting parallel lines ___ inches apart, using a top-to-bottom orientation, ___ out of ___ times.

29. Participate in a ___ *(School-Related Activity)* activity for ___ *(number)* minutes, with ___ *(number)* rest periods.

*30. Form horizontal lines moving from left to right, ___ out of ___ times, with verbal cues only.

*31. Draw ___ *(number)* circles between parallel lines which are ___ inches apart, using counterclockwise orientation, ___ out of ___ times.

*32. Draw ___ *(number)* crossed lines between parallel lines which are ___ inches apart, using top-to-bottom, left-to-right orientation, ___ out of ___ times.

(continued)

* These objectives are skills to be observed within the classroom setting. They may be especially useful in the total team-generated IEP models.

Graphomotor
  a. manuscript
  b. cursive
  c. upper
  d. lower
  e. A to Z

NOTES

*33. Form left-top-to-right-bottom and right-top-to-left-bottom diagonal lines, ___ out of ___ times, with verbal cues only.

*34. Form ___ *(upper/lower)*-case letter ___ *(A to Z)* in ___ *(manuscript/cursive)* writing, using correct directionality of letter formation, ___ out of ___ times, after demonstration.

*35. Copy ___ *(upper/lower)*-case letter ___ *(A to Z)* in ___ *(manuscript/cursive)* writing, using correct directionality of letter formation, ___ out of ___ times.

*36. Copy the letters ___ *(A to Z)* with proper formation, orientation, and closure, ___ out of ___ times.

*37. On request, form ___ *(upper/lower)*-case letter ___ *(A to Z)* in ___ *(manuscript/cursive)* writing, using correct directionality of letter formation, ___ out of ___ times.

*38. Uniformly space letters, words, and/or sentences when writing, ___% of the time.

Customized objectives:

* These objectives are skills to be observed within the classroom setting. They may be especially useful in the total team-generated IEP models.

Graphomotor
  a. manuscript
  b. cursive
  c. upper
  d. lower
  e. A to Z

NOTES

Long-Term Goal 7

To improve visual perception and/or perceptual motor skills for greater success in academics and written work.

Objective D

To demonstrate improved visual sequencing and visual memory, _____(child's name) will:

*1. Indicate which one of ___ (number) objects or pictures has been removed, after viewing for ___ (number) seconds.

*2. Look at a picture and immediately recall ___ (number) details.

*3. Look at a picture, and after a ___ (number)-second delay, recall ___ (number) details.

4. Imitate correctly a ___ (number)-part sequence of silent finger tapping immediately after presentation, ___ out of ___ times.

*5. Duplicate the correct sequence of a ___ (number)-part visual stimulus immediately after having viewed the model for ___ (number) seconds, ___ out of ___ times.

*6. Copy ___ (number) letters from a page, using not more than ___ (number) visual fixations, ___ out of ___ times.

*7. Copy ___ (number) words from a sentence, using not more than ___ (number) visual fixations, ___ out of ___ times.

*8. Form ___ (upper/lower)-case letter ___ (A to Z) in ___ (manuscript/cursive) writing, using correct directionality of letter formation, after demonstration, ___ out of ___ times.

*9. On request, form ___ (upper/lower)-case letter ___ (A to Z) in ___ (manuscript/cursive) writing, using correct directionality of letter formation, ___ out of ___ times.

*10. Uniformly space letters, words, and/or sentences when writing, ___% of the time.

*11. Copy a sentence with attention to details of letters, spacing, and punctuation, with fewer than ___ (number) omissions or errors.

Customized objectives:

* These objectives are skills to be observed within the classroom setting. They may be especially useful in the total team-generated IEP models.

Long-Term Goal 7

To improve visual perception and/or perceptual motor skills for greater success in academics and written work.

Objective E

To demonstrate improved visual figure ground abilities, _____(child's name) will:

*1. Locate ___ (number) named objects in the classroom environment, within ___ (number) seconds.

*2. Find a named object among a collection of objects, within ___ (number) seconds.

*3. Find a named object among a collection of similar objects, within ___ (number) seconds.

*4. Find a presented or named picture among a collection of pictures, within ___ (number) seconds.

*5. Find a presented or named shape among a collection of shapes, within ___ (number) seconds.

*6. Find a presented or named number or letter among a collection of numbers or letters, within ___ (number) seconds.

*7. Identify ___ (number) out of ___ (number) pictures hidden within the background of a picture, within ___ (number) seconds.

*8. Identify ___ (number) out of ___ (number) numbers hidden within the background of a picture, within ___ (number) seconds.

*9. Identify ___ (number) out of ___ (number) letters hidden within the background of a picture, within ___ (number) seconds.

*10. Identify a letter or shape which has been outlined in dotted lines, within ___ (number) seconds, ___ out of ___ times.

*11. Demonstrate visual closure in tasks such as forming circles, letters, and numbers, ___ out of ___ times.

Customized objectives:

* These objectives are skills to be observed within the classroom setting. They may be especially useful in the total team-generated IEP models.

QUALIFIERS

Graphomotor
  a. manuscript
  b. cursive
  c. upper
  d. lower
  e. A to Z

NOTES

Long-Term Goal 7

To improve visual perception and/or perceptual motor skills for greater success in academics and written work.

Objective F

To demonstrate improved discrimination of the visual properties of objects or pictures, _____(child's name) will:

*1. Arrange graduated or nesting objects by size, within ___ (number) minute(s).

*2. Identify between big and little, ___ out of ___ times.

*3. Differentiate big, medium, and little, ___ out of ___ times.

*4. Identify between tall and short, ___ out of ___ times.

*5. Identify between longer and shorter, ___ out of ___ times.

*6. Indicate which stimulus is in a different spatial orientation from the other ___ (number) presented, ___ out of ___ times.

*7. Identify what letter or shape has been outlined in dotted lines, within ___ (number) seconds, ___ out of ___ times.

*8. Demonstrate visual closure in tasks such as forming circles, letters, and numbers, ___ out of ___ times.

*9. Color a simple ___-inch shape, within ___ inch(es) of the boundary.

*10. Color an area not larger than 2 inches, using only finger movements, ___% of the time.

*11. Draw ___ (number) vertical lines connecting two parallel lines which are ___ inch(es) apart, using only isolated finger movements, ___ out of ___ times.

*12. Draw ___ (number) circles between two parallel lines which are ___ inch(es) apart, using only isolated finger movements, ___ out of ___ times.

*13. Draw ___ (number) connected loops between two parallel lines which are ___ inch(es) apart, using only isolated finger movements, ___ out of ___ times.

*14. Trace ___-inch high ___ (upper/lower)-case letter(s) ___ (A to Z), using ___ (manuscript/cursive) writing, within ___-inch accuracy.

Customized objectives:

* These objectives are skills to be observed within the classroom setting. They may be especially useful in the total team-generated IEP models.

Long-Term Goal 7

To improve visual perception and/or perceptual motor skills for greater success in academics and written work.

Objective G

To demonstrate improved visual closure abilities, _____(*child's name*) will:

*1. Identify a letter or shape which has been outlined in dotted lines, within ___ *(number)* seconds, ___ out of ___ times.

*2. Mentally complete circles, letters, and/or numbers, given only minimal outlines, ___ out of ___ times.

Customized objectives:

* These objectives are skills to be observed within the classroom setting. They may be especially useful in the total team-generated IEP models.

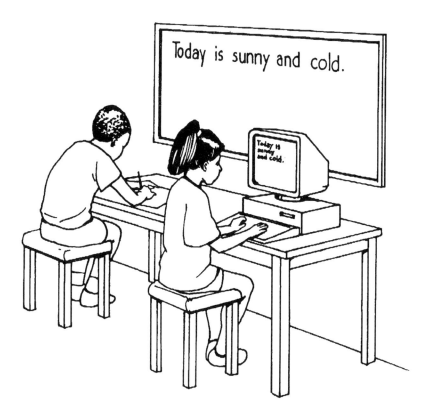

LONG-TERM GOAL
8

To improve written communication skills for greater proficiency when using writing implements and/or a keyboard.

QUALIFIERS

Plane
   a. horizontal
   b. vertical
   c. diagonal
   d. circular
   e. rotary
   f. pendular
   g. linear
   h. forward
   i. backward
   j. sideways
   k. forward, backward, and sideways
   l. multidirectional

Shapes
   a. vertical line
   b. horizontal line
   c. circle
   d. crossed lines
   e. X
   f. square
   g. triangle
   h. vertical diamond
   i. horizontal diamond

NOTES

Long-Term Goal 8

To improve written communication skills for greater proficiency when using writing implements and/or a keyboard.

Objective A

To demonstrate motor control needed for prewriting tasks, _____(child's name) will:

*1. Imitate a recognizable ___ (Shape) in a ___ (Plane) plane, ___ out of ___ times.

*2. Color a simple ___-inch shape, within ___ inch(es) of the boundary in a ___ (Plane) plane.

*3. Draw a straight line, within a ___-inch wide path without touching sides for a distance of ___ inches in a ___ (Plane) plane.

*4. Draw a line, within a ___-inch wide 5-inch long, horizontal S-curved path without touching the sides in a ___ (Plane) plane.

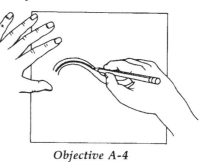

Objective A-4

*5. Use wrist movements to vary the direction of strokes when coloring, rather than turning the paper, ___% of the time.

*6. Trace along a ___-inch (Shape), with ___-inch accuracy in a ___ (Plane) plane.

*7. Trace along a ___-inch zigzag line consisting of ___ (number) diagonals, with ___-inch accuracy in a ___ (Plane)

*8. Connect ___ (number) dots which are ___ (number) inches apart, using straight lines, within ___-inch accuracy from the side of the dots in a ___ (Plane) plane.

*9. Color an area not larger than 2 inches, using only finger movements, ___% of the time.

Objective A-7

Customized objectives:

---

* These objectives are skills to be observed within the classroom setting. They may be especially useful in the total team-generated IEP models.

Graphomotor
  a. manuscript
  b. cursive
  c. upper
  d. lower
  e. A to Z

      NOTES

Long-Term Goal 8

To improve written communication skills for greater proficiency when using writing implements and/or a keyboard.

Objective B

To demonstrate intrinsic muscle control for pencil manipulation, _____ (child's name) will:

1. Hold pencil in the air with tripod grasp and walk fingers up and down pencil shaft, ___ (number) times, using ___ (number) steps.

2. Hold pencil in air with tripod grasp and fully rotate so that markings on pencil shaft move in a clockwise and then counterclockwise direction, ___ (number) consecutive times each.

3. Twirl pencil in a complete circular pattern, passing it end-over-end using only thumb, index, and middle fingers, ___ (number) consecutive times.

Objective B-2

*4. Reposition pencil from writing position to erasing position, using only one hand, ___ out of ___ times.

*5. Draw ___ (number) vertical lines connecting two parallel lines which are ___ inch(es) apart, using only isolated finger movements, ___ out of ___ times.

*6. Draw ___ (number) circles between two parallel lines which are ___ inch(es) apart, using only isolated finger movements, ___ out of ___ times.

*7. Draw ___ (number) connected loops between two parallel lines which are ___ inch(es) apart, using only isolated finger movements, ___ out of ___ times.

*8. Use isolated finger movements to write the alphabet in ___ (upper/lower)-case ___ (manuscript/cursive) writing, for ___ (number) of the 26 letters.

Customized objectives:

* These objectives are skills to be observed within the classroom setting. They may be especially useful in the total team-generated IEP models.

QUALIFIERS

School-Related Activities
  a. physical education
  b. playground
  c. classroom
  d. fine motor
  e. gross motor
  f. postural
  g. desk top
  h. (any specific activity
     of your choice)

Graphomotor
  a. manuscript
  b. cursive
  c. upper
  d. lower
  e. A to Z

NOTES

Long-Term Goal 8

To improve written communication skills for greater proficiency when using writing implements and/or a keyboard.

Objective C

To demonstrate motor control necessary for writing tasks, _____(child's name) will:

*1. Grade pressure applied when writing or coloring so as not to break the implement or wrinkle or rip the paper, ___% of the time.

*2. Erase pencil markings without wrinkling or ripping the paper, ___% of the time.

*3. Draw ___ (number) vertical lines connecting two parallel lines which are ___ inch(es) apart, within ___-inch accuracy.

*4. Draw ___ (number) vertical lines connecting parallel lines ___ inch(es) apart, using a top-to-bottom orientation, ___ out of ___ times.

*5. Participate in a ___ (School-Related Activity) activity for ___ (number) minutes, with ___ (number) rest periods.

*6. Draw ___ (number) out of ___ (number) vertical lines, using a top-to-bottom orientation, in order to connect two parallel lines ___ inches apart, within ___-inch accuracy.

*7. Draw ___ (number) circles between two parallel lines which are ___ (number) inch(es) apart, touching both top and bottom lines, with ___-inch accuracy.

*8. Draw ___ (number) circles between parallel lines which are ___ inches apart, using counterclockwise orientation, ___ out of ___ times.

*9. Draw ___ (number) crossed lines between parallel lines which are ___ inches apart, using top-to-bottom, left-to-right orientation, ___ out of ___ times.

*10. Trace ___-inch high ___ (upper/lower)-case letter(s) ___ (A to Z), using ___ (manuscript/cursive) writing, within ___-inch accuracy.

*11. Form ___ (upper/lower)-case letter(s) ___ (A to Z) in ___ (manuscript/ cursive) writing, using correct directionality of letter formation, after demonstration, ___ out of ___ times.

*12. Copy ____ (upper/lower)-case letter(s) ___ (A to Z) in ____ (manuscript/ cursive) writing, using correct directionality of letter formation, ___ out of ___ times.

(continued)

* These objectives are skills to be observed within the classroom setting. They may be especially useful in the total team-generated IEP models.

Duration
  a. seconds
  b. minutes
  c. repetitions

Graphomotor
  a. manuscript
  b. cursive
  c. upper
  d. lower
  e. A to Z

NOTES

Long-Term Goal 8, Objective C (continued)

*13. Copy ___ *(A to Z)* legibly, within ___ *(number) (Duration)*.

*14. Copy the letter(s) ___ *(A to Z)* with proper formation, orientation, and closure, ___ out of ___ times.

*15. Form ___ *(upper/lower)*-case letter(s) ___ *(A to Z)* on request in ___ *(manuscript/cursive)* writing, using correct directionality of letter formation, ___ out of ___ times.

*16. Uniformly space letters, words, and/or sentences when writing, ___% of the time.

*17. Copy a sentence with attention to details of letters, spacing, and punctuation, with fewer than ___ *(number)* omissions or errors.

Customized objectives:

* These objectives are skills to be observed within the classroom setting. They may be especially useful in the total team-generated IEP models.

Long-Term Goal 8

To improve written communication skills for greater proficiency when using writing implements and/or a keyboard.

Objective D

To demonstrate motor control necessary for using classroom tools associated with the pencil, _____(child's name) will:

*1. Completely erase pencil markings without wrinkling or ripping the paper, ___% of the time.

*2. Use a manual classroom pencil sharpener effectively and efficiently, ___% of the time.

*3. Hold a ruler in place while drawing a straight line along the ruler edge, with fewer then ___ (number) slips.

*4. Hold a stencil in place while drawing along the stencil edges, with fewer then ___ (number) slips.

*5. Use a ___ (Classroom Tool) effectively and efficiently, ___% of the time.

Customized objectives:

---

* These objectives are skills to be observed within the classroom setting. They may be especially useful in the total team-generated IEP models.

Degree of Assistance
  a. minimum(ly)
  b. moderate(ly)
  c. maximum(ly)
  d. verbal
  e. hand-over-hand
  f. physical
  g. tactile
  h. auditory
  i. visual
  j. no
  k. (any combination of above)

Type of Assistance
  a. assistance
  b. supervision
  c. guidance
  d. prompt
  e. demonstration
  f. cues
  g. in functional activities
  h. independently
  i. with gravity (assisted)
  j. gravity eliminated
  k. against gravity
  l. with ___ facilitation to ___
  m. with adapted devices
  n. passive
  o. active
  p. adaptive techniques
  q. (any combination of above)

Duration
  a. seconds
  b. minutes
  c. repetitions

NOTES

Long-Term Goal 8

To improve written communication skills for greater proficiency when using writing implements and/or a keyboard.

Objective E

To demonstrate motor control necessary for effective use of a keyboard, _____(child's name) will:

*1. Isolate fingers, within ___ (number) seconds, ___% of the time, to depress specific keys, using a hunt-and-peck technique.

*2. Isolate fingers, within ___ (number) seconds, ___% of the time, to depress specific keys, using the touch typing technique.

*3. Isolate fingers to depress specific keys, using the touch-typing technique with minimal glances at keys, ___% of the time.

*4. Recall ___ (number) letters or words with one visual fixation on material being copied.

*5. Coordinate fingers to desired keys in order to type ___ (number) letters/words per minute.

*6. Coordinate fingers to desired keys in order to type the alphabet in less than ___ (number) ___ (Duration).

*7. Maintain elbows at sides and use only wrist and finger movements when depressing the keys, ___ out of ___ times observed.

*8. Utilize compensatory techniques and/or adaptive equipment to depress keys, ___ out of ___ times observed.

*9. Turn on computer and/or printer, insert disc, use Save and Print functions, and begin keyboarding with ___ (Degree of Assistance) ___ (Type of Assistance).

*10. Turn on computer and/or printer, insert disc, and use Save and Print functions, and begin keyboarding independently, ___ out of ___ times.

Customized objectives:

* These objectives are skills to be observed within the classroom setting. They may be especially useful in the total team-generated IEP models.

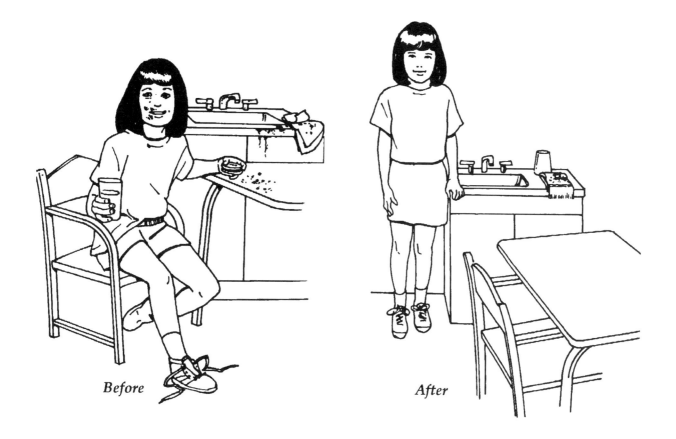

Before

After

LONG-TERM GOAL
9

To improve self-care skills for greater independence in school and home environments.

QUALIFIERS

Degree of Assistance
a. minimum(ly)
b. moderate(ly)
c. maximum(ly)
d. verbal
e. hand-over-hand
f. physical
g. tactile
h. auditory
i. visual
j. no
k. (any combination of above)

Type of Assistance
a. assistance
b. supervision
c. guidance
d. prompt
e. demonstration
f. cues
g. in functional activities
h. independently
i. with gravity (assisted)
j. gravity eliminated
k. against gravity
l. with ___ facilitation to ___
m. with adapted devices
n. passive
o. active
p. adaptive techniques
q. (any combination of above)

Hand/Foot Usage
a. preferred
e. right
f. left

NOTES

Long-Term Goal 9

To improve self-care skills for greater independence in school and home environments.

Objective A

To demonstrate functional lunch and snack skills, _____(*child's name*) will:

*1. With ___ *(Degree of Assistance)* ___ *(Type of Assistance)*, successfully use a spoon, ___% of the time.

*2. With ___ *(Degree of Assistance)* ___ *(Type of Assistance)*, sip a drink from a cup or glass, ___% of the time.

*3. With ___ *(Degree of Assistance)* ___ *(Type of Assistance)*, successfully use a fork, ___% of the time.

*4. With ___ *(Degree of Assistance)* ___ *(Type of Assistance)*, use a knife for spreading, ___% of the time.

*5. With ___ *(Degree of Assistance)* ___ *(Type of Assistance)*, use a knife for cutting, ___% of the time.

*6. With ___ *(Degree of Assistance)* ___ *(Type of Assistance)*, use adaptive equipment needed to accomplish task, ___% of the time.

*7. With ___ *(Degree of Assistance)* ___ *(Type of Assistance)*, carry mealtime items, ___% of the time.

*8. With ___ *(Degree of Assistance)* ___ *(Type of Assistance)*, pour liquids without spilling, ___% of the time.

*9. With ___ (Degree of Assistance) ___ (Type of Assistance), open packages and containers, ___% of the time.

*10. With ___ *(Degree of Assistance)* ___ *(Type of Assistance)*, follow mealtime routine, ___% of the time.

*11. Exhibit socially acceptable behaviors while eating, ___% of the time.

*12. Exhibit socially acceptable performance while eating, ___% of the time.

*13. Carry mealtime tray with ___ *(Hand/Foot Usage)* hand(s) successfully.

Customized objectives:

---

* These objectives are skills to be observed within the classroom setting. They may be especially useful in the total team-generated IEP models.

QUALIFIERS

Degree of Assistance
   a. minimum(ly)
   b. moderate(ly)
   c. maximum(ly)
   d. verbal
   e. hand-over-hand
   f. physical
   g. tactile
   h. auditory
   i. visual
   j. no
   k. (any combination of above)

Type of Assistance
   a. assistance
   b. supervision
   c. guidance
   d. prompt
   e. demonstration
   f. cues
   g. in functional activities
   h. independently
   i. with gravity (assisted)
   j. gravity eliminated
   k. against gravity
   l. with ___ facilitation to ___
   m. with adapted devices
   n. passive
   o. active
   p. adaptive techniques
   q. (any combination of above)

Dressing
   a. coats/sweaters
   b. hat
   c. gloves/mittens
   d. boots
   e. shoes
   f. socks
   g. button-down smock/shirt
   h. pullover smock/shirt
   i. belt
   j. braces/orthotics
   k. clothes

Fasteners
a. large buttons
b. small buttons
c. separating zipper
d. nonseparating zipper
e. snaps
f. buckle
g. Velcro®

Velcro® is a registered trademark of Velcro U.S.A., Inc.

Long-Term Goal 9

To improve self-care skills for greater independence in school and home environments.

Objective B

To demonstrate functional dressing skills, _____(child's name) will:

*1. With ___ (Degree of Assistance) ___ (Type of Assistance), remove ___ (Dressing), ___% of the time.

*2. With ___ (Degree of Assistance) ___ (Type of Assistance), put on ___ (Dressing), ___% of the time.

*3. With ___ (Degree of Assistance) ___ (Type of Assistance), adjust clothing for toileting, ___% of the time.

*4. With ___ (Degree of Assistance) ___ (Type of Assistance), put on ___ (Dressing) in the appropriate orientation, ___% of the time.

*5. With ___ (Degree of Assistance) ___ (Type of Assistance), open a ___ (Fastener), ___% of the time.

*6. With ___ (Degree of Assistance) ___ (Type of Assistance), close a ___ (Fastener), ___% of the time.

*7. With ___ (Degree of Assistance) ___ (Type of Assistance), untie shoelaces, ___% of the time.

*8. With ___ (Degree of Assistance) ___ (Type of Assistance), tie shoelaces in a bow, ___% of the time.

*9. With ___ (Degree of Assistance) ___ (Type of Assistance), lace shoes accurately, ___% of the time.

*10. With ___ (Degree of Assistance) ___ (Type of Assistance), use adaptive technique or device to put on ___ (Dressing).

*11. With ___ (Degree of Assistance) ___ (Type of Assistance), use adaptive technique or device to put on ___ (Dressing).

*12. With ___ (Degree of Assistance) ___ (Type of Assistance), adjust ___ (Dressing) appropriately to maintain a socially acceptable appearance, ___% of the time.

*13. With ___ (Degree of Assistance) ___ (Type of Assistance), use adaptive techniques or device to manipulate ___ (Fastener), ___% of the time.

*14. Assume responsibility for appropriate personal appearance and hygiene with ___ (Degree of Assistance) ___ (Type of Assistance), ___% of the time.

Customized objectives:

* These objectives are skills to be observed within the classroom setting. They may be especially useful in the total team-generated IEP models.

Degree of Assistance
a. minimum(ly)
b. moderate(ly)
c. maximum(ly)
d. verbal
e. hand-over-hand
f. physical
g. tactile
h. auditory
i. visual
j. no
k. (any combination of above)

Type of Assistance
a. assistance
b. supervision
c. guidance
d. prompt
e. demonstration
f. cues
g. in functional activities
h. independently
i. with gravity (assisted)
j. gravity eliminated
k. against gravity
l. with ___ facilitation to ___
m. with adapted devices
n. passive
o. active
p. adaptive techniques
q. (any combination of above)

NOTES

Long-Term Goal 9

To improve self-care skills for greater independence in school and home environments.

Objective C

To demonstrate functional hygiene and grooming skills, _____(child's name) will:

*1. With ___ (Degree of Assistance) ___ (Type of Assistance), use tissue to wipe nose, ___% of the time.

*2. With ___ (Degree of Assistance) ___ (Type of Assistance), indicate need to use toilet, ___% of the time.

*3. With ___ (Degree of Assistance) ___ (Type of Assistance), get on and off toilet, ___% of the time.

*4. With ___ (Degree of Assistance) ___ (Type of Assistance), use toilet, ___% of the time.

*5. With ___ (Degree of Assistance) ___ (Type of Assistance), turn water on and off, ___% of the time.

*6. With ___ (Degree of Assistance) ___ (Type of Assistance), adjust water temperature, ___% of the time.

*7. With ___ (Degree of Assistance) ___ (Type of Assistance), adjust water pressure, ___% of the time.

*8. With ___ (Degree of Assistance) ___ (Type of Assistance), wash hands and face thoroughly, ___% of the time.

*9. With ___ (Degree of Assistance) ___ (Type of Assistance), dry hands and face thoroughly, ___% of the time.

*10. With ___ (Degree of Assistance) ___ (Type of Assistance), exhibit socially acceptable hair care, ___% of the time.

*11. With ___ (Degree of Assistance) ___ (Type of Assistance), exhibit socially acceptable and appropriate behaviors and appearance, ___% of the time.

*12. Assume responsibility for appropriate personal appearance and hygiene, with ___ (Degree of Assistance) ___ (Type of Assistance), ___% of the time.

Customized objectives:

* These objectives are skills to be observed within the classroom setting. They may be especially useful in the total team-generated IEP models.

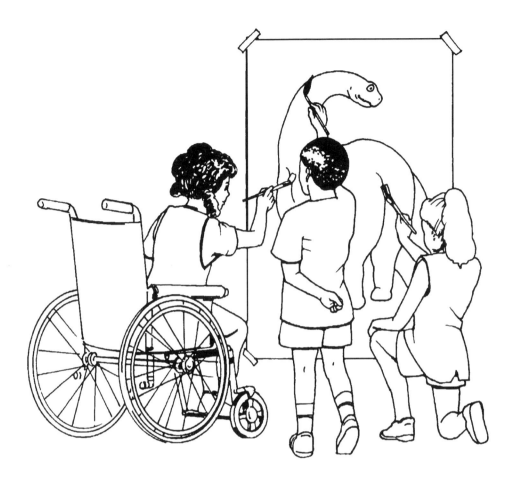

LONG-TERM GOAL
10

To improve work behaviors for greater task orientation in the classroom or vocational environment.

Long-Term Goal 10

To improve work behaviors for greater task orientation in the classroom or vocational environment.

Objective A

To demonstrate the ability to cooperatively function within a group, _____ (child's name) will:

*1. With ___ (Degree of Assistance) ___ (Type of Assistance), participate in a ___ (Size) group activity, ___% of the time.

*2. With ___ (Degree of Assistance) ___ (Type of Assistance), take turns as the rules require, ___% of the time.

*3. With ___ (Degree of Assistance) ___ (Type of Assistance), share materials, ___% of the time.

*4. With ___ (Degree of Assistance) ___ (Type of Assistance), change working roles as needed to complete a group activity, ___% of the time.

*5. Exhibit socially acceptable behaviors while eating, ___% of the time.

*6. Exhibit socially acceptable performance while eating, ___% of the time.

Customized objectives:

* These objectives are skills to be observed within the classroom setting. They may be especially useful in the total team-generated IEP models.

Long-Term Goal 10

To improve work behaviors for greater task orientation in the classroom or vocational environment.

Objective B

To demonstrate functional attending skills, _____(child's name) will:

*1. With ___ *(Degree of Assistance)* ___ *(Type of Assistance)*, maintain visual focus on task for ___ *(number)* ___ *(Duration)*, ___% of the time.

*2. With ___ *(Degree of Assistance)* ___ *(Type of Assistance)*, maintain socially acceptable eye contact with peers and authority figures, ___% of the time.

*3. With ___ *(Degree of Assistance)* ___ *(Type of Assistance)*, sit for ___ *(number)* ___ *(Duration)* during a classroom or school activity, ___% of the time.

*4. With ___ *(Degree of Assistance)* ___ *(Type of Assistance)*, follow a ___ *(number)*-step direction, ___% of the time.

Customized objectives:

* These objectives are skills to be observed within the classroom setting. They may be especially useful in the total team-generated IEP models.

QUALIFIERS

Degree of Assistance
  a. minimum(ly)
  b. moderate(ly)
  c. maximum(ly)
  d. verbal
  e. hand-over-hand
  f. physical
  g. tactile
  h. auditory
  i. visual
  j. no
  k. (any combination of above)

Type of Assistance
  a. assistance
  b. supervision
  c. guidance
  d. prompt
  e. demonstration
  f. cues
  g. in functional activities
  h. independently
  i. with gravity (assisted)
  j. gravity eliminated
  k. against gravity
  l. with ___ facilitation to ___
  m. with adapted devices
  n. passive
  o. active
  p. adaptive techniques
  q. (any combination of above)

NOTES

Long-Term Goal 10

To improve work behaviors for greater task orientation in the classroom or vocational environment.

Objective C

To demonstrate effective self-coping skills, _____(child's name) will:

*1. With ___ *(Degree of Assistance)* ___ *(Type of Assistance)*, cooperate when demands and requests are made, ___% of the time.

*2. Identify self by name, upon request, ___% of the time.

*3. With ___ *(Degree of Assistance)* ___ *(Type of Assistance)*, display orientation to familiar places within the environment, ___% of the time.

*4. With ___ *(Degree of Assistance)* ___ *(Type of Assistance)*, demonstrate the ability to navigate to familiar places within the environment, ___% of the time.

*5. With ___ *(Degree of Assistance)* ___ *(Type of Assistance)*, assume responsibility for appropriate personal appearance and hygiene, ___% of the time.

*6. Participate in activities and tasks which are perceived as unfamiliar or challenging, ___% of the time.

*7. Accept ___ *(Degree of Assistance)* assistance during an activity as needed, ___% of the time.

*8. With ___ *(Degree of Assistance)* ___ *(Type of Assistance)*, adhere to rules and regulations, ___% of the time.

*9. Seek assistance only after making an effort to independently perform the task, ___% of the time.

*10. Seek assistance when necessary, ___% of the time.

*11. Exhibit tolerance and respect for authority, ___% of the time.

*12. With ___ *(Degree of Assistance)* ___ *(Type of Assistance)*, show physical and verbal respect for others, ___% of the time.

*13. Accept demonstration and instruction before or during an activity, ___% of the time.

*14. Willingly change tasks, ___% of the time.

*15. With ___ *(Degree of Assistance)* ___ *(Type of Assistance)*, stay on task until it is completed, ___% of the time.

(continued)

* These objectives are skills to be observed within the classroom setting. They may be especially useful in the total team-generated IEP models.

Long-Term Goal 10, Objective C (continued)

*16. With ___ (Degree of Assistance) ___ (Type of Assistance), exhibit a positive verbal or physical response after completing a task, ___% of the time.

*17. With ___ (Degree of Assistance) ___ (Type of Assistance), maneuver through the environment while maintaining self, materials, and surroundings, ___% of the time.

*18. With ___ (Degree of Assistance) ___ (Type of Assistance), persevere in difficult activities, exhibiting a functional level of frustration tolerance, ___% of the time.

*19. With ___ (Degree of Assistance) ___ (Type of Assistance), persevere in difficult activities, ___% of the time.

*20. With ___ (Degree of Assistance) ___ (Type of Assistance), wait for instructor's attention during an activity, ___% of the time.

*21. With ___ (Degree of Assistance) ___ (Type of Assistance), gather necessary materials for an activity or task, ___% of the time.

*22. Assume responsibility for actions, ___% of the time.

*23. With ___ (Degree of Assistance) ___ (Type of Assistance), assume responsibility for personal belongings, including location and condition, ___% of the time.

*24. Make a decision, within ___ (number) seconds when given a choice of ___ (number) alternatives.

*25. Maintain socially acceptable eye contact with peers and authority figures with ___ (Degree of Assistance) ___ (Type of Assistance), ___% of the time.

*26. With ___ (Degree of Assistance) ___ (Type of Assistance), direct negative feelings toward task rather than at self or others, ___% of the time.

*27. With ___ (Degree of Assistance) ___ (Type of Assistance), express frustration and/or negative feelings in a socially accepted manner, ___% of the time.

*28. With ___ (Degree of Assistance) ___ (Type of Assistance), display good sportsmanship, ___% of the time.

*29. With ___ (Degree of Assistance) ___ (Type of Assistance), identify ___ (number) strengths and ___ (number) weaknesses of self.

*30. With ___ (Degree of Assistance) ___ (Type of Assistance), indicate awareness of limitations and strengths by making appropriate choices or judgments regarding participation in activities, ___% of the time.

(continued)

* These objectives are skills to be observed within the classroom setting. They may be especially useful in the total team-generated IEP models.

QUALIFIERS

Degree of Assistance
a. minimum(ly)
b. moderate(ly)
c. maximum(ly)
d. verbal
e. hand-over-hand
f. physical
g. tactile
h. auditory
i. visual
j. no
k. (any combination of above)

Type of Assistance
a. assistance
b. supervision
c. guidance
d. prompt
e. demonstration
f. cues
g. in functional activities
h. independently
i. with gravity (assisted)
j. gravity eliminated
k. against gravity
l. with ___ facilitation to ___
m. with adapted devices
n. passive
o. active
p. adaptive techniques
q. (any combination of above)

NOTES

*31. Participate in activities with a functional level of self-esteem and self-confidence, ___% of the time.

*32. Accept constructive criticism and feedback, ___% of the time.

*33. With ___ *(Degree of Assistance)* ___ *(Type of Assistance)*, exhibit assertive behaviors to protect self from physical and emotional harm and to maintain self-rights, ___% of the time.

*34. With ___ *(Degree of Assistance)* ___ *(Type of Assistance)*, follow a ___ *(number)*-step direction, ___% of the time.

Customized objectives:

* These objectives are skills to be observed within the classroom setting. They may be especially useful in the total team-generated IEP models.

Long-Term Goal 10

To improve work behaviors for greater task orientation in the classroom/vocational environment.

Objective D

To demonstrate effective task coping skills, _____ (child's name) will:

*1. With ___ (Degree of Assistance) ___ (Type of Assistance), follow a ___ (number)-step direction, ___% of the time.

*2. With ___ (Degree of Assistance) ___ (Type of Assistance), follow procedures of the classroom or work place, ___% of the time.

*3. With ___ (Degree of Assistance) ___ (Type of Assistance), locate necessary materials to complete a task, ___% of the time.

*4. With ___ (Degree of Assistance) ___ (Type of Assistance), exhibit functional organization of materials to complete a given activity in the allotted time, ___% of the time.

*5. Exhibit functional organization during a given task by maintaining the condition of all materials and the surrounding environment, ___% of the time.

*6. With ___ (Degree of Assistance) ___ (Type of Assistance), complete a given task within ___ minutes, ___% of the time.

*7. With ___ (Degree of Assistance) ___ (Type of Assistance), complete a given task, with attention to all necessary details, ___% of the time.

*8. With ___ (Degree of Assistance) ___ (Type of Assistance), complete a given task, attending to neatness and details, ___% of the time.

*9. Complete a given work assignment, attending to neatness and details, within ___ minutes, ___% of the time.

*10. With ___ (Degree of Assistance) ___ (Type of Assistance), complete work assignments with a consistent level of speed and accuracy, ___% of the time.

*11. Correct error(s) on own initiative, within ___ (number) seconds of having made the error(s), ___ out of ___ times.

*12. With ___ (Degree of Assistance) ___ (Type of Assistance), follow mealtime routine, ___% of the time.

*13. With ___ (Degree of Assistance) ___ (Type of Assistance), share materials, ___% of the time.

(continued)

* These objectives are skills to be observed within the classroom setting. They may be especially useful in the total team-generated IEP models.

*14. With ___ *(Degree of Assistance)* ___ *(Type of Assistance)*, change working roles as needed to complete a group activity, ___% of the time.

*15. Participate in activities and tasks which are perceived as unfamiliar or challenging, ___% of the time.

*16. Accept ___ *(Degree of Assistance)* assistance during an activity as needed, ___% of the time.

*17. With ___ *(Degree of Assistance)* ___ *(Type of Assistance)*, adhere to rules and regulations, ___% of the time.

*18. Seek assistance only after making an effort to perform the task, ___% of the time.

*19. Seek assistance when necessary, ___% of the time.

*20. Exhibit tolerance and respect for authority, ___% of the time.

*21. Participate in a ___ *(School-Related Activity)* activity for ___ minutes, with ___ *(number)* rest periods.

Customized objectives:

* These objectives are skills to be observed within the classroom setting. They may be especially useful in the total team-generated IEP models.

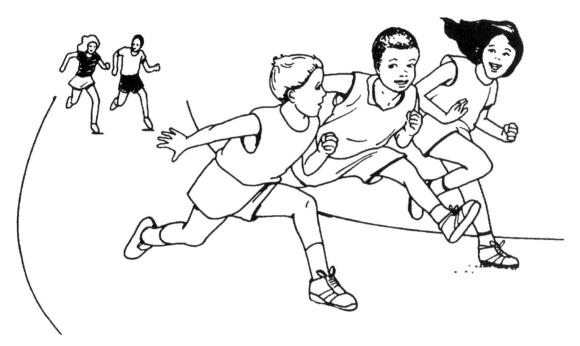

LONG-TERM GOAL
11

To improve or sustain participation in a task or activity for an age-appropriate length of time.

School-Related Activities

a. physical education
b. playground
c. classroom
d. fine motor
e. gross motor
f. postural
g. desk top
h. (any specific activity
   of your choice)

NOTES

Long-Term Goal 11

To improve or sustain participation in a task or activity for an age-appropriate length of time.

Objective

To demonstrate improved endurance, _____(*child's name*) will:

*1. Participate in a physical education activity for ___ minutes, with ___ (*number*) rest periods.

*2. Participate in a classroom activity for ___ minutes, with ___ (*number*) rest periods.

*3. Participate in a desk-top activity for ___ minutes, with ___ (*number*) rest periods.

*4. Participate in a writing activity for ___ minutes, with ___ (*number*) rest periods.

*5. Participate in a playground activity for ___ minutes, with ___ (*number*) rest periods.

*6. Participate in a ___ (*School-Related Activity*) activity for ___ minutes, with ___ (*number*) rest periods.

Customized objectives:

* These objectives are skills to be observed within the classroom setting. They may be especially useful in the total team-generated IEP models.

ADDITIONAL MATERIAL

CASE STUDIES

Occupational therapy services can be provided in many ways, including direct services (center-based, school-based, home-based), school and home consultation, transdisciplinary consultation, and monitoring. The goals and objectives and methods and strategies should reflect the model that is being used.

The case studies in this chapter are but a few examples of the practical applications of *OT GOALs*. The types of goals and the models of service delivery are determined by the needs of the child, family, and/or school. Although *OT GOALs* allows for individualization of goals, objectives, methods, and strategies, additional ones may need to be developed to address the individuality of each child.

CASE STUDY #1—PETER

Peter is a four-year, two-month-old boy who attends a local integrated preschool. He was referred for an occupational therapy evaluation by his teacher, who stated concerns in the areas of behavior and motor skills. He reported that Peter prefers to play alone. Although Peter plays within the proximity of other children, he becomes aggressive when children get too close to him. Peter's teacher reports that he has difficulty drawing shapes and skillfully manipulating toys like the other children his age. He stated that Peter "is often tripping over his own two feet."

During the occupational therapy evaluation, Peter demonstrated an appropriate concentration/attention span in a structured situation. He attempted and persisted with all tasks presented to him. However, Peter's play style tended to be rigid and somewhat ritualistic.

Peter presented with deficits in sensory motor processing. This was evidenced by his lack of smooth, binocular visual tracking, the presence of tactile defensiveness, and poor tactile discrimination. He also had a hyporesponsive postrotary nystagmus following rotation or spinning activities. Peter did not have a consistent eye-hand-foot dominance. He did not appear to have good coordination between the two sides of his body.

Peter presented with poor postural control secondary to low muscle tone. He had difficulty with movements and positions against gravity, such as supine flexion and prone extension, and his preferred floor-sitting position was W-sitting. He presented with decreased shoulder stability in both weight-bearing and nonweight-bearing positions. Peter lacked midrange control when reaching for objects in space, and he used immature grasp-and-release patterns. Subsequently, Peter's fine motor and visual motor scores were delayed.

Peter's self-help skills were mildly delayed. He was able to put on and take off his pants, shirt, socks, coat, mittens, and hat; but he had difficulty with fastenings.

The occupational therapy evaluation summary indicated that Peter had a sensory integration deficit. His inability to process and organize sensory input (such as touch, vision, and movement) were impacting on his behavior and motor skills in the classroom.

Following the occupational therapy evaluation, Peter's parents and team met to discuss his current needs. Goal areas were targeted. The following goals and objectives (see the worksheets on pages 144-145 and detail on pages 146-151) were formulated by the occupational therapist individually. However, these goals and objectives were directly related to Peter's classroom functioning.

OT GOALs WORKSHEET B

Occupational Therapy Goals and Objectives 19_93_ -19_94_

Name: _Peter_   Therapist: _N. Q., OTR_

Date: _9-13-93_   District: _New Town_

Code:
LTG = Long-Term Goal   # = Number of Objective
OBJ = Objective   Qualifiers = (Fill in from Qualifiers list)

Page _43_ LTG _1_ ; OBJ _A_ ; # _1_ ; Qualifiers _5 out of 5 times_ ;

Methods _1, 5, 17, 18_ ; Strategies _*, 16, 18, 20_ ; Materials _3_ ;

Who _1, 5, 4_ ; Evaluations _16, 1, 2, 7_
* Provide monitoring and collaborative consultation for teacher-implemented program

Page _43_ LTG _1_ ; OBJ _A_ ; # _3_ ; Qualifiers _50%_ ;

Methods _1, 5, 17, 18_ ; Strategies _*, 16, 18, 20_ ; Materials _3_ ;

Who _1, 4, 5_ ; Evaluations _16, 1, 2, 7_
* Provide monitoring and collaborative consultation for teacher-implemented program

Page _45_ LTG _1_ ; OBJ _C_ ; # _5_ ; Qualifiers _1_ ;

Methods _1, 5, 17, 18_ ; Strategies _*, 16, 18, 20_ ; Materials _3_ ;

Who _1, 4, 5_ ; Evaluations _16, 1, 2, 7_
* Provide monitoring and collaborative consultation for teacher-implemented program

Page _51_ LTG _2_ ; OBJ _A_ ; # _1_ ; Qualifiers _5_ ;

Methods _1, 5, 17, 18_ ; Strategies _5, 10, 13, 16_ ; Materials _1, 2, 26, 33;_
medium ball, 34-medium bolster, 36

Who _1, 4, 7_ ; Evaluations _1, 4, 7_

Page _51_ LTG _2_ ; OBJ _A_ ; # _5_ ; Qualifiers _10_ ;

Methods _1, 5, 17, 18_ ; Strategies _5, 10, 13, 16_ ; Materials _1, 2, 26,_ ;
33 - medium ball, 34 - medium bolster, 36

Who _1, 4, 7_ ; Evaluations _1, 4, 7_

Page _57_ LTG _3_ ; OBJ _A_ ; # _4_ ; Qualifiers _9 out of 10 times_ ;

Methods _1, 5_ ; Strategies _5, 7, 10, 11, 14, 15, 16, 31_ ; Materials _2, 4, 5, 6, 13, 14, 25, 28, 3, 31_

Who _1, 4, 5_ ; Evaluations _1, 4_

see page 2

SAMPLE WORKSHEET (continued)

OT GOALs WORKSHEET B

Occupational Therapy Goals and Objectives 19_____-19_____

Name: *Peter* _____ Therapist: _____

Date: _____ District: _____

Code:
LTG = Long-Term Goal   # = Number of Objective
OBJ = Objective   Qualifiers = (Fill in from Qualifiers list)

Page __58__ LTG __3__; OBJ __B__; # __2__; Qualifiers _small, 9 out of 10 times_;
Methods __1, 5__; Strategies _5, 7, 10, 11, 14, 15, 16, 31_; Materials _14, 25, 28, 3, 2, 4, 5, 6, 13, 31_
Who __1, 4, 5__; Evaluations __1, 4__

Page __59__ LTG __3__; OBJ __C__; # __9__; Qualifiers _10 out of 10 times_;
Methods __1, 5__; Strategies _5, 7, 10, 11, 14, 15, 16, 31_; Materials _14, 25, 28, 3, 2, 4, 5, 6, 13, 31_
Who __1, 4, 5__; Evaluations __1, 4__

Page __59__ LTG __3__; OBJ __C__; # __10__; Qualifiers __25__;
Methods __1, 5__; Strategies _5, 7, 10, 11, 14, 15, 16, 31_; Materials _25, 28, 3, 31, 2, 4, 5, 6, 13, 14_
Who __1, 4, 5__; Evaluations __1, 4__

Page __60__ LTG __3__; OBJ __D__; # __1__; Qualifiers _9, 5 out of 10 times_;
Methods __1, 5__; Strategies _5, 7, 10, 11, 14, 15, 16, 31_; Materials _25, 28, 3, 31, 2, 4, 5, 6, 13, 14_
Who __1, 4, 5__; Evaluations __1, 4__

Page __62__ LTG __3__; OBJ __F__; # __9__; Qualifiers _10_;
Methods __1, 5__; Strategies _5, 7, 10, 11, 14, 15, 16, 31_; Materials _25, 28, 3, 31, 2, 4, 5, 6, 13, 14_
Who __1, 4, 5__; Evaluations __1, 4__

Page __n/a__ LTG __3__; OBJ __H__; # __*__; Qualifiers _____;
Methods __1, 5__; Strategies _5, 7, 10, 11, 14, 15, 16, 31_; Materials _25, 28, 3, 31, 2, 4, 5, 6, 13, 14_
Who __1, 4, 5__; Evaluations __1, 4__

* To demonstrate isolated finger control, Peter will manipulate all fasteners during dressing tasks.

CASE STUDY #1—PETER

INSTRUCTIONAL GUIDE

Peter
September 13, 1993

Long-Term Goal 1:
To improve ability to use sensory information to understand and effectively interact with people and objects in the school and home environments.

> *Objective:* To demonstrate improved accommodation to touch sensations, Peter will accept anticipated touch during a group activity, 100% of the time.

> *Objective:* To demonstrate improved accommodation to touch sensations, Peter will accept unexpected touch without behavioral over-reactions, 50% of the time.

> *Objective:* To demonstrate improved awareness and discrimination of touch sensations, Peter will point to the place on fingers that was touched lightly, when vision was occluded, within 1 centimeter of accuracy.

Methods:
1. Direct occupational therapist individual intervention

2. Occupational therapist consultation with the classroom teacher

3. Home-program suggestions

4. Parent/Caregiver intervention

Strategies:
1. Provide monitoring and collaborative consultation for teacher-implemented program.

2. Guide the child through the motions of a fine motor activity to provide tactile/proprioceptive and kinesthetic feedback.

3. Provide a multisensory approach as required.

4. Enhance the child's participation through high-interest activities.

Materials: Those used in tactile-stimulatory activities, such as:
Shaving cream

Finger paint

Clay dough

Peter
September 13, 1993
Instructional Guide (continued)

Who:
1. Occupational therapist

2. Classroom teacher

3. Parent/Caregiver

Evaluation:
1. Sensory testing

2. Occupational therapist's clinical observations

3. Classroom teacher's observations

4. Parent/Caregiver's observations

Long-Term Goal 2:
To improve postural control to provide a stable base of support needed to facilitate better hand use for manipulation of classroom materials, posture while working and playing, and mobility in the school and home environments.

Objective: To demonstrate improved balance between flexor and extensor musculature (cocontraction), Peter will maintain a lifted and extended posture of the head and upper body from a prone (on stomach) position, for 5 seconds.

Objective: To demonstrate improved balance between flexor and extensor musculature (cocontraction), Peter will maintain a lifted and curled position of the neck and shoulders, with arms crossed over the chest, from a supine (on back) position, for 10 seconds.

Methods:
1. Direct occupational therapist individual intervention

2. Occupational therapist consultation with the classroom teacher

3. Home-program suggestions

4. Parent/Caregiver intervention

Strategies:
1. Utilize therapeutic preparatory techniques, with ongoing use of these techniques as needed to facilitate adaptive responses.

2. Adapt fine motor activities as needed.

3. Provide practice and repetition to reinforce skill development.

4. Guide the child through the motions of a gross motor activity to provide tactile/proprioceptive and kinesthetic feedback.

Materials:

Suspended equipment, such as netswings, platform swing

Scooterboards

Obstacle courses

Medium-sized therapy ball

Medium-sized bolster

Balance-beam activities

Who:

1. Occupational therapist

2. Physical education teacher

3. Parent/Caregiver

Evaluation:

1. Occupational therapist's clinical observations

2. Physical education teacher's observations

3. Parent/Caregiver observations

Long-Term Goal 3:

To improve functional shoulder, arm, and hand control for greater success with fine motor tasks and classroom and home manipulatives

Objective: To demonstrate purposeful and accurate reach toward objects, Peter will use an appropriate reach pattern, 9 out of 10 times.

Objective: To demonstrate appropriate release patterns, Peter will utilize controlled release of an object above a small container with wrist extension, 9 out of 10 times.

Objective: To demonstrate appropriate grasp or pinch pattern, Peter will hold object between tips of opposed thumb and index finger (fine pincer), 10 out of 10 times.

Objective: To demonstrate appropriate grasp or pinch pattern, Peter will use a static tripod grasp when writing with a pencil, 75% of the time.

Objective: To demonstrate hand preference/dominance, Peter will reach for and grasp objects with preferred hand, 5 out of 10 times.

Objective: To demonstrate arm midrange control/grading of movement using appropriate force and accuracy, in order to perform physical education, art, and classroom activities with control and precision, Peter will stack 10 one-inch cubes without arm resting on table.

Objective: To demonstrate isolated finger control, Peter will manipulate all fasteners during dressing tasks.

Objective: To demonstrate improved arm strength and stability needed as a foundation for controlled movement, Peter will wheelbarrow walk for a distance of 10 feet, with support provided at the knees.

Methods:
1. Direct occupational therapist individual intervention
2. Occupational therapist consultation with the classroom teacher

Strategies:
1. Utilize therapeutic preparatory techniques, with ongoing use of these techniques as needed to facilitate adaptive responses.
2. Present fine motor activities in developmental sequence.
3. Adapt fine motor activities as needed.
4. Grade fine motor activities as needed.
5. Adjust the child's positioning to improve performance.
6. Provide positive reinforcement.
7. Guide child through the motions of a fine motor activity to provide tactile/proprioceptive and kinesthetic feedback.
8. Utilize upper-extremity weight-bearing activities.

Materials:
Scooterboards

Toys and materials requiring resistive squeeze and grasp, such as clay, water pistols, tongs, tweezers

Toys and materials with small pieces, such as pegs, beads for stringing

Playground equipment

Cut-and-paste activities

Coloring activities

Toys requiring twisting and untwisting

Paper-and-pencil mazes

Finger painting

Putty exercises

Who:
1. Occupational therapist
2. Classroom teacher
3. Parent/Caregiver

Evaluation:

1. Occupational therapist's clinical observations

2. Physical education teacher's observations

Long-Term Goal 4:

To improve ocular motor control for greater success in reading, writing, copying, and eye-hand coordination tasks

> *Objective:* To demonstrate visual tracking, Peter will use disassociated eye movements from the head to successfully follow a Wiffle® ball suspended from a 3-foot string as it swings horizontally at eye level, for 10 seconds.

Methods:

1. Direct occupational therapist individual intervention

2. Parent/Caregiver intervention

Strategies:

1. Provide practice and repetition to reinforce skill development.

2. Adjust the child's positioning to improve performance.

3. Enhance the child's participation through high-interest activities.

Materials:

Target games

Specialized computer software

Hidden-picture games

Who:

1. Occupational therapist

2. Parent/Caregiver

Evaluation:

1. Occupational therapist's clinical observations

2. Parent/Caregiver's observations

Long-Term Goal 5:

To improve written communication skills for greater proficiency when using writing implements and/or a keyboard

> *Objective:* To demonstrate motor control needed for prewriting tasks, Peter will imitate a circle and an X recognizably, 2 out of 3 times.

Wiffle® is a registered trademark of The Wiffle Ball, Inc., Shelton, CT.

Methods:
1. Direct individual intervention by occupational therapist

2. Occupational therapist consultation with the classroom teacher

3. Home-program suggestions

4. Parent/Caregiver intervention

Strategies:
1. Provide verbal cues as needed.

2. Provide demonstration as needed.

3. Provide hand-over-hand assistance.

4. Provide practice and repetition to reinforce skill development.

5. Guide child through motions of fine motor activity to provide tactile/proprioceptive and kinesthetic feedback.

6. Provide a multisensory approach as required.

7. Present visual motor activities in developmental sequence.

Materials:
Toys incorporating shape concepts

Scissor activities

Specialized computer software

Cut-and-paste activities

Coloring activities

Painting with assorted paintbrushes

Clay dough activities

Who:
1. Occupational therapist

2. Classroom teacher

3. Parent/Caregiver

Evaluation:
1. Occupational therapist's clinical observations

2. Classroom teacher's observations

3. Parent/Caregiver's observations

4. Visual-motor evaluation

CASE STUDY #2—LAURA

Laura is a five-year-old girl with a medical diagnosis of cerebral palsy, spastic diplegia. She has been receiving direct center-based occupational therapy services since the age of eight months. She recently received a yearly reevaluation to update her status and to set goals for the upcoming year. Parental concerns for her at this time include her awkward fine motor skills and her limited self-help/ADL skills.

During the occupational therapy reevaluation, Laura demonstrated good concentration and attention span. She attempted and persisted with all tasks presented to her, no matter how difficult the task.

Laura presented with adequate sensory motor responses, which included good oculomotor control, refined tactile discrimination, and accurate awareness of limb positions and movements. She enjoyed both self-initiated and imposed movements during scooterboard, netswing, and therapy ball activities.

Laura demonstrated moderately increased extensor and adductor tone in both lower extremities. This increased muscle tone causes her legs to be very stiff and in an excessively straight position. It is difficult for her to keep her legs apart, which causes her feet to hit each other while she walks. She wears bilateral ankle-foot orthoses and ambulates with a posterior walker. Muscle tone in her trunk and upper extremities was low. Passive range of motion was full throughout upper and lower limbs, trunk, and pelvis. Laura maintained short-sitting in an adapted chair independently. In short-sitting, however, her pelvis was posteriorly tilted, her back was rounded, and her shoulders were in a position of internal rotation and protraction. Active reach was limited to 120 degrees of shoulder flexion and abduction; subsequently, her pectoral muscles were tight due to muscle shortening.

Laura lacked many of the motor components required for age-appropriate fine-motor skills. Her reaching patterns tended to be in a pronated fashion (palm side of hand facing down), thus limiting her view of objects in her hands. Her reach lacked smooth control and she frequently overshot or undershot her target. Grasp patterns were delayed. She used an inferior pincer grasp of small objects (thumb against the side of the index finger instead of the tip), and a digital pronate grasp of a pencil (pencil held with the thumb and all fingers instead of a three-finger grasp).

Release of objects in a variety of sizes and shapes was accomplished by using wrist flexion and/or surface contact (for example, bending the wrist down to straighten the fingers, or pressing the object against a surface to assist in release). Laura had much difficulty isolating finger movements, and she had poor manipulation of objects within her hand. Fine motor skills and visual-motor integration, as measured by appropriate assessment tools, were two years delayed.

Visual-perceptual skills (nonmotor) also were assessed. This was an area of strength for Laura; she presented with age-appropriate skills in all areas.

Laura demonstrated difficulties in the areas of self-help/ADL. She was unable to put on or take off elastic-waist pants or a pullover shirt. She was able to put on or take off her coat, hat, and gloves, but not her shoes, socks, or braces. She was not able to manipulate fasteners such as buttons, snaps, and hooks. Laura was independent in toileting and most grooming and hygiene tasks; however, she had much difficulty washing, combing, and styling her hair due to upper-extremity reaching limitations.

After reviewing the findings of the occupational therapy reevaluation with Laura and her family, goal areas were jointly developed. The following goals and objectives (see the worksheets on pages 155-156 and detail on pages 157-162) were developed from that process.

SAMPLE WORKSHEET FOR CASE #2

OT GOALs WORKSHEET B

Occupational Therapy Goals and Objectives 19_93_ -19_94_

Name: _Laura_   Therapist: _M. G. – OTR_

Date: _9-30-93_   District: _New Town_

Code:
LTG = Long-Term Goal   # = Number of Objective
OBJ = Objective   Qualifiers = (Fill in from Qualifiers list)

Page _52_   LTG _2_ ; OBJ _A_ ; # _12*_ ; Qualifiers _10 minutes_ ;

Methods _1, 17, 18, 11_ ; Strategies _5, 13, 15, 14_; Materials _6, 7, 33, 34_;

Who _1, 2, 4_ ; Evaluations _1, 7_
* *"Upper extremity"* – not arms ; classroom activity – not fine motor

Page _59_   LTG _3*_ ; OBJ _C_ ; # _8_ ; Qualifiers _8/10_ ;

Methods _1, 17, 18_ ; Strategies _5, 7, 13, 15, 16, 10_ ; Materials _4, 5, 31_ ;

Who _1, 4_ ; Evaluations _1, 7_   potty exercise

* To improve upper extremity control and fine motor skills to enhance classroom performance.

Page _75_   LTG _3_ ; OBJ _N_ ; # _6_ ; Qualifiers _—_ ;

Methods ____ ; Strategies ____ ; Materials ____ ;

Who ____ ; Evaluations ____

Page _62_   LTG _3_ ; OBJ _F_ ; # _9_ ; Qualifiers _5_ ;

Methods ____ ; Strategies ____ ; Materials ____ ;

Who ____ ; Evaluations ____

Page _62_   LTG _3_ ; OBJ _F_ ; # _7_ ; Qualifiers _6, 3/4 w/out resting hand or arm on table_ ;

Methods ____ ; Strategies ____ ; Materials ____ ;

Who ____ ; Evaluations ____

Page _66_   LTG _3_ ; OBJ _N_ ; # _2_ ; Qualifiers _25%_ ;

Methods ____ ; Strategies ____ ; Materials ____ ;

Who ____ ; Evaluations ____

Please list all these objectives, then list all methods, strategies, etc.

see page 2

SAMPLE WORKSHEET (continued)

OT GOALs WORKSHEET B

Occupational Therapy Goals and Objectives 19_____-19_____

Name: _Laura_____   Therapist: _____

Date: _____   District: _____

Code:
LTG = Long-Term Goal   # = Number of Objective
OBJ = Objective   Qualifiers = (Fill in from Qualifiers list)

See note on p. 1

Page _66_ LTG _3_; OBJ _A_; # _1_; Qualifiers _75%_____;

Methods _____; Strategies _____; Materials _____;

Who_____; Evaluations _____

Page _66_ LTG _3_; OBJ _A_; # _10_; Qualifiers _index; 3/4_____;

Methods _____; Strategies _____; Materials _____;

Who_____; Evaluations _____

Page _66_ LTG _3_; OBJ _A_; # _3_; Qualifiers _3/4_____;

Methods _1, 11, 17, 18_; Strategies _4, 5, 7, 13, 14_; Materials _4, 5, 12, 13, 14_;

Who_ 1, 4 _; Evaluations _13, 1_

Page _124_ LTG _9_; OBJ _B_; # _5_; Qualifiers _j, a, g   75%____;

Methods _____; Strategies _____; Materials _____;

Who_____; Evaluations _____

Page _124_ LTG _9_; OBJ _B_; # _6_; Qualifiers _j, a, g   75%____;

Methods _____; Strategies _____; Materials _____;

Who_____; Evaluations _____

Page _124_ LTG _9_; OBJ _B_; # _13_; Qualifiers _j, a, d   75%____;

Methods _1, 17, 18_; Strategies _15, 19, 26_ [2, 3, 4, 12, 13, 14]; Materials _20, Clothing w/ Velcro closing_;

Who_ 1, 4, 5 _; Evaluations _1, 7, 2_

Again, list all objectives - then materials, methods, etc.

CASE STUDY #2—LAURA

GOALS AND OBJECTIVES

Laura
September 30, 1993

Long-Term Goal 1:

To improve postural control to provide a stable base of support needed to facilitate better hand use for manipulation of classroom materials, posture while working, and mobility in the home and school environments.

> *Objective:* To demonstrate improved balance between flexor and extensor musculature, Laura will maintain a functional sitting posture with upright head and trunk, hips at 90 degrees and feet flat on the floor, without support of the upper extremities, during classroom activities, while positioned in an adaptive chair, for 10 minutes.

Methods:

1. Direct service occupational therapy

2. Home-program suggestions

3. Parent/Caregiver intervention

4. Occupational therapy consultation with the physical therapist

Strategies:

1. Utilize therapeutic preparatory techniques, with ongoing use of these as needed to facilitate adaptive responses.

2. Provide practice and repetition to reinforce skill development.

3. Vary the child's positioning to improve performance.

4. Provide positive reinforcement.

Materials:

Playground equipment

Adaptive equipment

Therapy balls in small, medium, and large sizes

Bolsters in small, medium, and large sizes

Who:

1. Occupational therapist

2. Physical therapist

3. Parent/Caregiver

Laura
September 30, 1993
Goals and Objectives (continued)

Evaluation:
1. Occupational therapist's clinical observations

2. Parent/Caregiver's observations

Long-Term Goal 2:
To improve upper-extremity control and fine motor skills to enhance classroom performance

> *Objective:* To demonstrate appropriate grasp or pinch pattern, Laura will hold object between pads of the opposed thumb and index finger with thumb and finger slightly flexed (neat pincer), 8 out of 10 times.

Methods:
1. Direct service occupational therapy

2. Home-program suggestions

3. Parent/Caregiver intervention

Strategies:
1. Utilize therapeutic preparatory techniques, with ongoing use of these techniques as needed to facilitate adaptive responses.

2. Present fine motor activities in developmental sequence.

3. Provide practice and repetition to reinforce skill development.

4. Provide positive reinforcement.

5. Guide the child through the motions of a fine motor activity to provide tactile/proprioceptive and kinesthetic feedback.

6. Adapt fine motor activities as needed.

Materials:
Toys and materials requiring resistive grasp and squeeze, such as putty, water pistols, tongs, tweezers

Toys and materials with small pieces, such as pegs, beads for stringing

Clay dough activities

Putty exercises

Who:
1. Occupational therapist

2. Parent/Caregiver

Evaluation:
1. Occupational therapist's clinical observations

2. Parent/Caregiver's observations

Laura
September 30, 1993
Goals and Objectives (continued)

Long-Term Goal 3:
To improve functional shoulder, arm, and hand control for greater success with fine motor tasks and classroom manipulatives

Objective: To maintain or improve functional range of motion, Laura will extend involved arm(s) over head, as in raising hand to answer question.

Objective: To maintain or improve functional range of motion, Laura will place hands behind her neck with elbows out to the side (for example, to adjust collar).

Objective: To demonstrate upper-extremity midrange control/grading of movement, in order to perform gym, art, and classroom activities with appropriate force and accuracy, Laura will stack 5 one-inch cubes without arm resting on table.

Objective: To demonstrate upper-extremity midrange control/grading of movement, in order to perform gym, art, and classroom activities with appropriate force and accuracy, Laura will place 6 large-sized pegs directly into a board without undershooting or overshooting the holes, 3 out of 4 times without resting arm or hand on table.

Objective: To demonstrate isolated finger control, Laura will point or poke with index finger, keeping all other fingers flexed, 75% of the time.

Objective: To demonstrate isolated finger control, Laura will extend each finger consecutively, as in counting, 75% of the time.

Objective: To demonstrate isolated finger control, Laura will depress intended keyboard characters with only index finger extended, 3 out of 4 times.

Objective: To demonstrate isolated finger control, Laura will trace desired form with one extended finger, keeping all others flexed, 3 out of 4 times.

Methods:
1. Direct service occupational therapy

2. Occupational therapy consultation with the physical therapist

3. Home-program suggestions

4. Parent/Caregiver intervention

Laura
September 30, 1993
Goals and Objectives (continued)

Strategies:

1. Provide hand-over-hand assistance.

2. Utilize therapeutic preparatory techniques, with ongoing use of these techniques as needed to facilitate adaptive responses.

3. Present fine motor activities in developmental sequence.

4. Provide practice and repetition to reinforce skill development.

5. Vary the child's positioning to improve performance.

Materials:

Toys and materials requiring resistive grasp and squeeze, such as putty, water pistols, tongs, tweezers

Toys and materials with small pieces, such as pegs

Stringing toys (beads, macaroni, sewing cards, spools)

Cut-and-paste activities

Coloring activities

Who:

1. Occupational therapist

2. Parent/Caregiver

Evaluation:

1. Goniometric evaluation

2. Occupational therapist's clinical observations

Long-Term Goal 4:

To improve written communication skills for greater proficiency when using writing implements and/or a keyboard

> *Objective:* To demonstrate motor control needed for prewriting tasks, Laura will use wrist movements to vary the direction of strokes when coloring, rather than turning the paper, 75% of the time.

Methods:

1. Direct service occupational therapy

2. Home-program suggestions

3. Parent/Caregiver intervention

Strategies:
1. Provide verbal cues as needed.

2. Provide demonstration as needed.

3. Provide hand-over-hand assistance.

4. Utilize therapeutic preparatory techniques, with ongoing use of these techniques as needed to facilitate adaptive responses.

5. Provide practice and repetition to reinforce skill development.

6. Vary the child's positioning to improve performance.

7. Guide the child through the motions of a fine motor activity to provide tactile/proprioceptive and kinesthetic feedback.

8. Provide a multisensory approach as required.

9. Utilize experimental learning techniques.

10. Provide adaptive equipment as needed.

Materials:
Adaptive equipment

Dress-up costumes

Who:
1. Occupational therapist

2. Parent/Caregiver

Evaluation:
1. Occupational therapist's clinical observations

2. Appropriate fine motor evaluation

3. Parent/Caregiver's observations

Long-Term Goal 5:
To improve self-care skills for greater independence in school and home environments.

Objective: To demonstrate functional dressings skills, Laura will open a Velcro® fastener with no assistance, 75% of the time.

Objective: To demonstrate functional dressing skills, Laura will close a Velcro® fastener with no assistance, 75% of the time.

Objective: To demonstrate functional dressing skills, Laura will use an adaptive technique/device to manipulate a nonseparating zipper, with no assistance, 75% of the time.

Velcro® is a registered trademark of Velcro U.S.A., Inc.

Laura
September 30, 1993
Goals and Objectives (continued)

Methods:
1. Direct service occupational therapy

2. Home-program suggestions

3. Parent/Caregiver intervention

Strategies:
1. Provide verbal cues as needed.

2. Provide demonstration as needed.

3. Provide hand-over-hand assistance.

4. Teach compensatory techniques.

5. Provide practice and repetition to reinforce skill development.

6. Vary the child's positioning to improve performance.

7. Provide positive reinforcement.

8. Require the child to specify an organizational plan before the task is implemented.

9. Provide adaptive equipment as needed.

Materials:
1. Dress-up costumes

2. Clothing with Velcro® closing

Who:
1. Occupational therapist

2. Parent/Caregiver

3. Teacher

Evaluation:
1. Occupational therapist's observations

2. Parent's/Caregiver's report

3. Teacher's observation

Velcro® is a registered trademark of Velcro U.S.A., Inc.

CASE STUDY #3—KELLY

Kelly is a three-year-old female with a diagnosis of Down syndrome. She entered her local preschool program after receiving three years of early intervention services. Kelly received an occupational therapy evaluation in her school to determine current related service needs and to provide input to the classroom teacher.

Kelly was attentive throughout the evaluation session. She followed simple directions well, and she attempted and persisted with all activities presented. She demonstrated good concentration and attention span.

Kelly presented with good sensory motor responses in visual, tactile, proprioceptive, kinesthetic, and vestibular (body awareness) skills. She enjoyed a variety of tactile activities, such as finger painting, play with foam, and beanbox play. She responded well to both imposed and self-initiated movement activities, such as being on a scooterboard, in a netswing, and on a therapy ball.

Kelly demonstrated low muscle tone throughout. However, she was able to move through all transitional positions, including sitting, kneeling, half-kneeling, standing, and running. Gross motor skills were near age level, with the exception of one-foot balance and hopping. Slight difficulties were noted with upper-extremity weight-bearing positions, such as wheelbarrow walking, propelling a scooterboard, and opening and closing classroom doors.

Kelly demonstrated functional reach and release skills. She demonstrated age-appropriate gross patterns, but grasp and pinch strength were weak. Isolated finger control, in-hand manipulation, and dexterity were slightly compromised, due to Kelly's tendency to use shoulder, wrist, and whole-hand manipulation during fine motor tasks. Subsequently, her fine motor and perceptual motor skills were delayed but approximated her cognitive level of 30 months. This was evidenced by difficulties using scissors, imitating strokes and designs with a crayon, removing a small cap from a bottle, completing a formboard, and unbuttoning large buttons.

Kelly had difficulties in the areas of self-help. Although she was able to remove all clothing, she was unable to put on a pullover shirt, elastic-waist pants, coat, hat, and gloves. She had much difficulty with all fastenings. In the areas of feeding, Kelly was able to finger feed, use a sipper cup, and use a fork. She was unable to use a regular cup or to spoon feed due to spillage. She was dependent in all areas of grooming and hygiene.

Evaluation results indicated the need for occupational therapy services. Following the Individualized Education Plan meeting, the team recommended an initial period of direct service occupational therapy, to set up a classroom program with the teacher and to investigate the need for adaptive techniques and equipment for self-help skills. Once this program is established, consultation should be provided at the teacher's request to adapt and/or modify Kelly's program. The team determined goals together. However, the goals were not stated in behavioral terms. The following goals and objectives (see the worksheets on pages 165-166 and detail on pages 167-170) were formulated by the occupational therapist to support the team's goals.

SAMPLE WORKSHEET FOR CASE #3

OT GOALs WORKSHEET B

Occupational Therapy Goals and Objectives 19 93 -19 94

Name: Kelly

Therapist: M. S. - OTR

Date: 1-10-94

District: Washington

Code:
LTG = Long-Term Goal
OBJ = Objective

\# = Number of Objective
Qualifiers = (Fill in from Qualifiers list)

Page 124   LTG 9 ; OBJ B ; # 4 ; Qualifiers a, pants, 100% ;
Methods 1, 5, 7, 17, 18, 3 ; Strategies 1, 2, 3, 4, 12, 13, 15, 16 ; Materials 20, oversized clothing; toys requiring twisting and untwisting
Who 1, 5, 9, 4 ; Evaluations 1, 2, Classroom paraprofessional's clinical observations, 7

Page 124   LTG 9 ; OBJ B ; # 4 ; Qualifiers j, a, a, 100% ;
Methods _____ ; Strategies _____ ; Materials _____ ;
Who _____ ; Evaluations _____

Page 123   LTG 9 ; OBJ a ; # 1 ; Qualifiers a, 75% ;
Methods _____ ; Strategies _____ ; Materials _____ ;
Who _____ ; Evaluations _____

Page 125   LTG 9 ; OBJ C ; # 8 ; Qualifiers d, f, 100% ;
Methods _____ ; Strategies _____ ; Materials _____ ;
Who _____ ; Evaluations _____

Page 125   LTG 9 ; OBJ C ; # 9 ; Qualifiers d, f, 100% ;
Methods _____ ; Strategies _____ ; Materials _____ ;
Who _____ ; Evaluations _____

Continue the same methods, strategies, materials, who, & evaluations for these.

Page 65   LTG 3 ; OBJ b ; # 11 ; Qualifiers 10, g ;
Methods 1, 5, 7, 3 ; Strategies 2, 3, 5, 6, 7, 15, 31 ; Materials 2, 4, 8, 13, 17, 16, 6, 31 ;
Who 1, 5, 9, 4 ; Evaluations 1, 2, 9

see page 2

SAMPLE WORKSHEET (continued)

OT GOALs WORKSHEET B

Occupational Therapy Goals and Objectives 19_____-19_____

Name: _Kelly_____   Therapist: _____

Date: _____   District: _____

Code:
LTG = Long-Term Goal   # = Number of Objective
OBJ = Objective   Qualifiers = (Fill in from Qualifiers list)

Page _65_ LTG _3_ ; OBJ _G_ ; # _15_ ; Qualifiers _____—_____ ;

Methods _____ ; Strategies _____ ; Materials _____

Who _____ ; Evaluations _____

Page _66_ LTG _3_ ; OBJ _H_ ; # _1_ ; Qualifiers _50%_ ;

Methods _____ ; Strategies _____ ; Materials _____

Who _____ ; Evaluations _____

Page _70_ LTG _3_ ; OBJ _G_ ; # _4_ ; Qualifiers _5_ ;

Methods _____ ; Strategies _____ ; Materials _____

Who _____ ; Evaluations _____

Page _71_ LTG _3_ ; OBJ _X_ ; # _2_ ; Qualifiers _10, a_ ;

Methods _____ ; Strategies _____ ; Materials _____

Who _____ ; Evaluations _____

Continue from methods on here.

Page _54_ LTG _2_ ; OBJ _C_ ; # _2_ ; Qualifiers _3 out of 4 times_ ;

Methods _1, 5, 17, 3_ ; Strategies _5, 6, 9, 15_ ; Materials _1, 6, 33, 36, 34_ ;

Who _1, 2, 5, 9, 4_ ; Evaluations _1, 2, 10, 18_

Page _54_ LTG _2_ ; OBJ _C_ ; # _10_ ; Qualifiers _a, 2_ ;

Methods _____ ; Strategies _____ ; Materials _____

Who _____ ; Evaluations _____

Continue from Methods w/ same as above

CASE STUDY #3—KELLY

GOALS AND OBJECTIVES

Kelly
January 10, 1994

Long-Term Goal 1:
To improve self-care skills for greater independence in school and home environments.

Objective: To demonstrate functional dressing skills, Kelly will put on pants in the appropriate orientation, with minimum assistance, 100% of the time.

Objective: To demonstrate functional dressing skills, Kelly will put on coat in the appropriate orientation, with no assistance, 100% of the time.

Objective: To demonstrate functional lunch and snack skills, Kelly will successfully use a spoon, with minimum assistance, 75% of the time.

Objective: To demonstrate functional hygiene and grooming skills, Kelly will wash hands and face thoroughly, with verbal cues, 100% of the time.

Objective: To demonstrate functional hygiene and grooming skills, Kelly will dry hands and face thoroughly, with verbal cues, 100% of the time.

Methods:
1. Individual occupational therapist intervention
2. Occupational therapist consultation with teacher and/or classroom paraprofessional
3. Home-program suggestions
4. Parent/Caregiver intervention
5. Occupational therapist monitoring

Strategies:
1. Provide minimal assistance.
2. Provide verbal cues as needed.
3. Provide demonstration as needed.
4. Provide hand-over-hand assistance.
5. Teach compensatory techniques where necessary.
6. Provide practice and repetition to reinforce skill development.
7. Provide positive reinforcement.
8. Guide the child through the motions of an activity to provide tactile/proprioceptive and kinesthetic feedback.

Kelly
January 10, 1994
Goals and Objectives (continued)

Materials:

Dress-up costumes

Oversized clothing

Toys requiring twisting and untwisting

Who:
1. Occupational therapist

2. Classroom teacher

3. Classroom paraprofessional

4. Parent/Caregiver

Evaluation:
1. Occupational therapist's clinical observations

2. Classroom teacher's clinical observations

3. Classroom paraprofessional's clinical observations

4. Parent/Caregiver's clinical observations

Long-Term Goal 2:

To improve functional shoulder, arm, and hand control for greater success with fine motor tasks and classroom manipulatives

Objective: To demonstrate improved arm strength and stability, needed as a foundation for controlled movement, Kelly will wheelbarrow walk for a distance of 10 feet, with support provided at the thighs.

Objective: To demonstrate improved arm strength and stability needed as a foundation for controlled movement, Kelly will independently push or pull open a school lavatory and/or exit door.

Objective: To demonstrate improved arm strength and stability needed as a foundation for controlled movement, Kelly will pull along a rope using a hand-over-hand pattern, while prone (on stomach) on a scooterboard, for a distance of 15 feet.

Objective: To demonstrate isolated finger control, Kelly will extend each finger consecutively, as in counting, 50% of the time.

Objective: To demonstrate prescissor skills, Kelly will use squeeze tongs to pick up and release 5 small objects.

Objective: To develop and refine scissor skills, using appropriate positioning, Kelly will snip edge of paper 10 times, using small classroom scissors.

Methods:

1. Individual occupational therapy intervention

2. Occupational therapist consultation with classroom teacher

3. Occupational therapist consultation with classroom paraprofessional

4. Occupational therapist monitoring

Strategies:

1. Provide verbal cues as needed.

2. Provide demonstration as needed.

3. Utilize therapeutic preparatory techniques, with ongoing use of these techniques as needed to facilitate adaptive responses.

4. Present gross motor activities in developmental sequence.

5. Present fine motor activities in developmental sequence.

6. Provide positive reinforcement.

7. Utilize upper-extremity weight-bearing activities.

Materials:

Scooterboard

Toys and materials requiring resistive grasp and squeeze such as clay, water pistols, tweezers

Puzzles

Cut-and-paste activities

Beanbags

Balls

Playground equipment

Clay dough activities

Who:

1. Occupational therapist

2. Classroom teacher

3. Classroom paraprofessional

4. Parent/Caregiver

Evaluation:

1. Occupational therapist's clinical observations

2. Classroom teacher's observations

3. Fine motor evaluation

Kelly
January 10, 1994
Goals and Objectives (continued)

Long-Term Goal 3:
To improve postural control to provide a stable base of support needed to facilitate better hand use for manipulation of classroom materials, posture while working, and mobility in school and home environments

Objective: To improve balance/equilibrium reactions, Kelly will respond with trunk, arm, and leg movement of one side when shifted to the opposite side, while half kneeling, 3 out of 4 times.

Objective: To improve balance/equilibrium reactions, Kelly will stand still on preferred foot, with eyes open and arms crossed over chest, for 2 seconds.

Methods:
1. Individual occupational therapy intervention
2. Occupational therapist consultation with classroom teacher and/or paraprofessional
3. Home-program suggestions
4. Occupational therapist monitoring

Strategies:
1. Utilize therapeutic preparatory techniques, with ongoing use of these techniques as needed to facilitate adaptive responses.
2. Present gross motor activities in developmental sequence.
3. Grade gross motor activities as needed.
4. Provide positive reinforcement.

Materials:
1. Suspended equipment, such as netswings, platform swing
2. Playground equipment
3. Therapy balls in small and medium sizes
4. Balance-beam activities
5. Medium-sized bolsters

Who:
1. Occupational therapist
2. Physical therapist
3. Classroom teacher/Paraprofessional
4. Parent/Caregiver

Evaluation:
1. Occupational therapist's clinical observations
2. Classroom teacher's observations
3. Gross motor evaluation
4. Standardized testing

CASE STUDY #4—CASEY

Casey is a seven-year-old boy in the second grade. He was referred for an occupational therapy evaluation due to handwriting problems. His teacher reported that he is very distractible and often has difficulty attending to tasks and completing activities.

During the occupational therapy evaluation, Casey was quite fidgety in his chair. He appeared to be distracted easily by visual and auditory stimulation. Although he was able to sit for long periods, it was difficult for him to focus on tasks presented.

Evaluation results indicated poor oculomotor control. He had much difficulty isolating eye movements during visual tracking. He was unable to perform saccadic eye movements (quick shifts of gaze) between two moving targets. Testing of vestibular functioning (response to movement stimulation), as measured by postrotary nystagmus following rotation, indicated a hyporesponsiveness to movement stimulation. He appeared to crave spinning movement; and, following this stimulation, he appeared to be calmer and more organized in his behavior and approach to tasks. Tactile, proprioceptive, and kinesthetic awareness (body awareness) responses were within normal limits.

Casey presented with the necessary motor components required for fine motor skills. These components included normal muscle tone and functional grasp, reach, and release patterns. However, due to Casey's difficulty in focusing on tasks, isolated finger movements were not well controlled, and he did not persist with activities long enough to use varied manipulation strategies.

Casey presented with global delays in the area of nonmotor visual perception. Subsequently, he had much difficulty with visual perceptual motor tasks, such as block and pegboard designs and design copying. Visual perceptual deficits also impacted on his cursive writing skills, as evidenced by poor spacing between letters and words. Letter sizes were distorted and letter formation was poor, lacking adequate directionality.

After reviewing the findings of the occupational therapy evaluation with Casey's parents and school team members, priorities were set for Casey's performance in school. The classroom teacher felt that he could address Casey's distractibility in the classroom, but he was interested in receiving input from the occupational therapist. Both Casey's parents and teacher wanted assistance with addressing handwriting difficulties. They wanted the final outcome to be that Casey would keep up with his classmates with written work. They were open to both remediation and/or compensation. To meet Casey's needs, the occupational therapist developed more specific goals and objectives for his educational plan. These included:

Objective: To demonstrate visual focusing skills, Casey will focus for 5 minutes on an object being held or manipulated.

This objective was added to the teacher's goals and objectives for promoting improved concentration and attention span.

The following long-term goals and objectives (see the worksheets on pages 172-173 and detail on pages 174-177) were added to Casey's IEP.

OT GOALs WORKSHEET A

Occupational Therapy Goals and Objectives 19_93_ -19_94_

Name: _Casey_   Therapist: _M. L. - OTR_

Date: _9-9-93_   District: _Washington_

Code:
LTG = Long-Term Goal
OBJ = Objective
# = Number of Objective
Qualifiers = (Fill in from Qualifiers list)

(1) Page _95_   LTG _6_ ; OBJ _a_ ; # _2_ _____ ; Qualifiers _5 minutes_

Page _96_   LTG _6_ ; OBJ _B_ ; # _10_ _____ ; Qualifiers _60 (each #)_

Page _96_   LTG _6_ ; OBJ _B_ ; # _5_ _____ ; Qualifiers _75%_

Page _96_   LTG _6_ ; OBJ _B_ ; # _9_ _____ ; Qualifiers _50%_

(2) Page _106_   LTG _7_ ; OBJ _C_ ; # _19_ _____ ; Qualifiers _1_

Page _106_   LTG _7_ ; OBJ _C_ ; # _25_ _____ ; Qualifiers _10 attempts_

Page _106_   LTG _7_ ; OBJ _C_ ; # _23_ _____ ; Qualifiers _others, 9/10_

(3) Page _118_   LTG _8_ ; OBJ _C_ ; # _16_ _____ ; Qualifiers _75%_

Page _118_   LTG _8_ ; OBJ _C_ ; # _15_ _____ ; Qualifiers _upper & lower, all, manuscript, 75%_

Page _118_   LTG ____ ; OBJ ____ ; # _____ ; Qualifiers _____

SAMPLE WORKSHEET (continued)

Methods	Strategies	Materials	Who	Evaluation
① 5, 1, 17, 18, 19, 20	① 15, 20, 21 mod, 22, 23 min, 29	① Classroom assignments 22, 23, 27, 28, 1	① 5, 1, 4	① 1, 2, 7
② 1, 5, 7, 18			② 1, 4, 5	② 11, 12, 1
	② 5, 13, 14	② 10, 11, 14, 15, 22, 27, 28, 29		
③ 1, 5, 18			③ 1, 4, 5	③ 1, 2, 7, 11, 12
	③ 2, 13, 18, 21 min, 22, 23 min, 24, 12	③ 7, 13, 14, 15, 22, 28, 29, 30, 31		

CASE STUDY #4—CASEY

GOALS AND OBJECTIVES

Casey
September 9, 1993

Long-Term Goal 1:
To improve ocular motor control for greater success in reading, writing, copying, and eye-hand coordination tasks

Objective: To demonstrate visual focusing skills, Casey will focus for 5 minutes on an object being held or manipulated.

Objective: To demonstrate visual tracking, Casey will follow the second hand of a classroom clock for 60 seconds, and correctly indicate as it passes over each number.

Objective: To demonstrate visual tracking, Casey will disassociate eye movements from the head during functional activities, 75% of the time.

Objective: To demonstrate visual tracking, Casey will maintain visual contact while the teacher is moving about the room, 50% of the time.

Long-Term Goal 2:
To improve perceptual motor skills for greater success in academics and written work

Objective: To demonstrate improved awareness of forms and spatial relations of objects to each other, Casey will copy age-appropriate cube designs with 1 attempt.

Objective: To demonstrate improved awareness of forms and spatial relations of objects to each other, Casey will join a picture which has been divided into 10 pieces.

Objective: To demonstrate improved awareness of forms and spatial relations of objects to each other, Casey will indicate which stimulus is in a different spatial orientation from the others presented, 9 out of 10 times.

Long-Term Goal 3:
To improve written communication skills for greater proficiency when using writing instruments and/or a keyboard

Objective: To demonstrate motor control necessary for writing tasks, Casey will uniformly space letters, words, and/or sentences when writing, 75% of the time.

Objective: To demonstrate motor control necessary for writing tasks, Casey will form all upper- and lower-case letters in manuscript writing, using correct directionality of letter formation, 75% of the time.

Methods:
Goal #1

a. Occupational therapy consultation with the classroom teacher

b. Individual occupational therapy intervention

c. Home-program suggestions

d. Parent/Caregiver intervention

e. Classroom teacher intervention

f. Special educator/Teacher intervention

Goal #2

a. Individual occupational therapy intervention

b. Occupational therapy consultation with classroom teacher

c. Occupational therapy consultation with the child's classroom paraprofessional

d. Parent/Caregiver intervention

Goal #3

a. Individual occupational therapy intervention

b. Occupational therapy consultation with the classroom teacher

c. Parent/Caregiver intervention

Strategies:
Goal #1

a. Provide positive reinforcement.

b. Enhance the child's participation through high-interest activities.

c. Provide moderate ongoing structure for task completion.

d. Provide decreasing structure for task completion.

e. Provide a work space with minimal distractions.

f. Utilize activities with increasing numbers of steps or sequences.

Goal #2

a. Utilize therapeutic preparatory techniques, with ongoing use of these techniques as needed to facilitate adaptive responses.

b. Provide practice and repetition to reinforce skill development.

c. Adjust the child's positioning to improve performance.

175

Goal #3

a. Provide verbal cues as needed.

b. Provide practice and repetition to reinforce skill development.

c. Provide a multisensory approach as required.

d. Provide minimal ongoing structure for task completion.

e. Provide decreasing structure for task completion.

f. Provide a workspace with minimal distractions.

g. Utilize experimental learning techniques.

h. Teach compensatory techniques.

Materials:
Goal #1

a. Classroom assignments

b. Specialized computer software

c. Board games

d. Hidden-picture games

e. Paper-and-pencil mazes

f. Suspended equipment, such as netswings, platform swing

Goal #2

a. Toys incorporating size concepts

b. Toys incorporating shape concepts

c. Coloring activities

d. Tracing activities

e. Specialized computer software

f. Hidden-picture games

g. Paper-and-pencil mazes

h. Dot-to-dot sheets

Goal #3

a. Adaptive equipment

b. Cut-and-paste activities

c. Coloring activities

d. Tracing activities

e. Specialized computer software

f. Paper-and-pencil mazes

g. Dot-to-dot sheets

h. Painting with assorted paintbrushes

i. Clay dough activities

Who:
Goal #1
a. Classroom teacher

b. Occupational therapist

c. Parent/Caregiver

Goal #2
a. Occupational therapist

b. Parent/Caregiver

c. Classroom teacher

Goal #3
a. Occupational therapist

b. Parent/Caregiver

c. Classroom teacher

Evaluation:
Goal #1
a. Occupational therapist's clinical observations

b. Classroom teacher's observations

c. Parent/Caregiver's observations

Goal #2
a. Appropriate visual-motor evaluation

b. Appropriate visual perception evaluation

c. Occupational therapist's clinical observations

Goal #3
a. Occupational therapist's clinical observations

b. Classroom teacher's observations

c. Parent/Caregiver's observations

d. Appropriate visual-motor evaluation

e. Appropriate visual perception evaluation

GLOSSARY

Abduction: Movement away from the body's midline.

Active range of motion: Self-imposed movement of a body part through the full excursion possible at a specific joint, using muscle contractions.

Adduction: Movement toward the body's midline.

Asymmetrical bilateral coordination: Simultaneously using both sides of the body to perform different movements.

Balance and equilibrium responses: Refers to many compensatory automatic movements used to regain midline stability; allows one to establish and re-establish one's center of gravity.

Bilateral coordination: Refers to smooth purposeful action of muscles on both sides of the body.

Cocontraction: Refers to the simultaneous activation of opposing muscle groups around the joint(s), resulting in stabilization or holding of a position at that point.

Crawl: Movement by pulling the body, using reciprocal arm and leg movements with belly touching floor.

Creep: Movement in a quadruped position by alternating arm and leg movements.

Directionality: The ability to perceive the directional relationship of object to self and/or another object.

Dynamic tripod pencil grasp: Holding pencil between pads of opposed thumb and index and side of middle finger's first joint, with ring and little finger flexed arching the palm. Writing by moving the fingers with the wrist slightly extended.

Extension: Straightening of a joint or a body part, using muscle contraction.

Extensor(s): Refers to the muscle(s) that straighten a joint or body part.

Fine pincer grasp: Holding an object between tips of opposed thumb and index finger.

Flexion: Bending a joint or part of the body, using muscle contraction.

Flexor(s): Refers to the muscle(s) that bend a joint or part of the body.

Half-kneel: Kneeling on one knee with other hip and knee flexed and foot flat on floor.

Hand dominance: Establishment or consistent use of a preferred hand, which becomes more skillful.

Inferior pincer grasp: Holding an object between the extended thumb and the index finger, proximal to the pad.

In-hand manipulation: Ability to hold an object and move it into different orientations, using only the thumb and fingers of one hand.

Intrinsic muscle control: Using the small muscles of the hand which are responsible for refined hand movements.

Isolated finger control: Ability to selectively move only a specified finger.

Kinesthesia: Refers to the awareness of joint movement through receptors in and around the joint.

Lateralization: The ability of the brain to process certain types of information on one side more efficiently than on the other side.

Lateral pinch grasp: Holding an object between adducted thumb and side of index finger.

Midline: Refers to an imaginary line through the center of the body from head to foot.

Midline crossing: Ability to reach across from the left side of the body to the right side of the body and vice versa.

Mid-range control: Ability to grade the movement between full extension and full flexion of specific muscle groups to smoothly perform an action.

Motor planning: Refers to one's ability to originate, plan, and execute a novel motor activity.

Neat pincer grasp: Holding an object between pads of opposed thumb and index finger, with finger and thumb slightly flexed.

Ocular motor control: Ability to coordinate the external muscles of the eye, producing smooth eye movements in all planes.

Opposition: Touching tips of thumb and finger(s) with rounded web space and slightly flexed fingers.

Passive range of motion: Body part is moved through the full excursion possible at a specific joint, with movement externally imposed.

180

Perception: Ability to perceive, organize, and act upon information received through the senses: seeing, hearing, smelling, tasting, touching, feeling movement, and position of the body in relation to self and to environment.

Perceptual motor: The ability to respond motorically to what is perceived.

Postural control: Refers to the skill required to maintain stability and alignment during daily activities.

Prone: Lying on stomach.

Proprioception: Refers to the awareness of the position of the body in space. Information is obtained from receptors in the muscles and joints.

Protective responses: Refers to extension of the extremities toward the supporting surface in response to sudden shift in the center of gravity.

Quadruped: Positioned with weight bearing only on hands and knees.

Radial digital grasp: Holding an object between opposed thumb and pads of fingers, with no palm involvement.

Radial palmar grasp: Flexion of fingers against an object pressing it into palm, with no thumb participation.

Reciprocal bilateral coordination: Using both sides of the body to perform the same movement in an alternating rhythmical pattern.

Side-sit: Sitting with weight primarily on one buttock, and hips and knees bent toward the weight-bearing side.

Spatial relations: Ability to see the position of objects in relation to self and in relation to each other.

Static pencil tripod grasp: Holding a pencil between pads of opposed thumb and index and side of middle finger's first joint, with ring and little fingers only slightly flexed. Writing occurs by moving the whole hand or arm, rather than the fingers.

Supine: Lying on back.

Symmetrical bilateral coordination: Performing the same action, using both sides of the body simultaneously.

Three-point grasp (tripod): Holding an object between pad of opposed thumb and pads of index and middle fingers.

Visual closure: Ability to mentally complete a letter, picture, or shape, given only a minimal outline.

Visual discrimination: Ability to see differences and similarities between stimuli.

Visual figure-ground: Ability to see and differentiate specific stimuli from background stimuli.

Visual fixation: Ability to focus eyes on stimulus for an appropriate length of time.

Visual localization: Ability to use quick, efficient eye movements to find specified stimuli.

Visual memory: Ability to see and remember a stimulus.

Visual sequencing: Ability to see and understand distinctions between objects or symbols, and to order them in a specified way.

Visual tracking: Ability to smoothly coordinate eye movements in various planes to follow a moving object.

Wheelbarrow walk: Walking on hands with elbows extended, and hips, knees, and/or ankles supported by someone else.

SUGGESTED READINGS

American Occupational Therapy Association. 1986. School occupational therapy survey. *AOTA Occupational Therapy News* 40(7):6.

_____. 1987. *Guidelines for Occupational Therapy Services in School Systems* (Revised). Rockville, MD: AOTA.

_____. 1989. *Guidelines for Occupational Therapy Services in Early Intervention and Preschool* (Revised). Rockville, MD: AOTA.

Ayres, A. J. 1972. *Sensory Integration and Learning Disorders.* Los Angeles: Western Psychological Services.

_____. 1980. *Sensory Integration and the Child.* Los Angeles: Western Psychological Services.

Bly, L. 1983. *The Components of Normal Development During the First Year of Life.* Chicago: Neurodevelopmental Treatment Associates Publishers.

Bobath, B. 1971. *Abnormal Postural Reflex Activity Caused by Brain Lesions.* London: William Heinemann Medical Books.

Bobath, B., and K. Bobath. 1975. *Motor Development in Different Types of Cerebral Palsy.* London: William Heinemann Medical Books.

Boehme, R. 1988. *Improving Upper Body Control.* Tucson, AZ: Therapy Skill Builders.

Brinckerhoff, J. L., and L. J. Vincent. 1986. Increasing parental decision making at the individualized educational program meeting. *Journal of the Division for Early Childhood* 11(1):46-58.

Caplan, F., and T. Caplan. 1977. *The Second Twelve Months of Life.* New York: Bantam Books, Inc.

_____. 1983. *The Early Childhood Years: The Two-Six Year Old.* New York: Bantam Books, Inc.

Clark, P. N., and A. S. Allen. 1985. *Occupational Therapy for Children* (Revised). St. Louis: C. V. Mosby Co.

DeQuiros, J., and O. Schrager. 1979. *Neuropsychological Fundamentals in Learning Disabilities.* San Rafael, CA: Academic Therapy.

Dunn, W. 1988. Models of occupational therapy service provision in the school system. *American Journal of Occupational Therapy* 42(11):718-723.

Erhardt, R. P. 1982. *Developmental Hand Dysfunction: Theory Assessment Treatment.* Baltimore: RAMSCO Publishers.

Fenton, K. S., R. Yoshida, J. P. Maxwell, and M. J. Kaufman. 1979. Recognition of team goals: An essential step toward rational decision making. *Exceptional Children* 45(8):638-644.

Finnie, N. R. 1975. *Handling the Young Cerebral Palsied Child.* New York: E. P. Dutton.

Giangreco, M. F. 1986. Delivery of therapeutic services in special education programs for learners with severe handicaps. *Physical and Occupational Therapy in Pediatrics* 6(2):5-15.

_____. 1990. Making related service decisions for students with severe disabilities: Roles, criteria, and authority. *Journal of the Association for Persons with Severe Handicaps* 15(1):22-31.

Giangreco, M. F., and B. Rainfroth. 1989. Providing related services to learners with severe handicaps in educational settings: Pursuing the least restrictive option. *Pediatric Physical Therapy* 1(2):55-63.

Gilfoyle, E., and C. Hays. 1979. Occupational therapy roles and functions in the education of the school-based handicapped student. *American Journal of Occupational Therapy* 33(9):565-576.

Gilfoyle, E., A. Grady, and T. Moore. 1981. *Children Adapt.* Thorofare, NJ: Charles B. Slack, Inc.

Ginburg, H., and S. Opper. 1979. *Piaget's Theory of Intellectual Development.* Englewood Cliffs, NJ: Prentice Hall, Inc.

Hopkins, H. L., and H. D. Smith. 1978. *Willard and Spackman's Occupational Therapy,* Fifth Ed. Philadelphia: J. B. Lippincott.

Knickerbocker, B. M. 1980. *A Holistic Approach to the Treatment of Learning Disorders.* Thorofare, NJ: Charles B. Slack, Inc.

McCormick, L., and C. Lee. 1979. P.L. 94-142: Mandated partnership. *American Journal of Occupational Therapy* 33(9):586-588.

Ottenbacher, K. 1983. Transdisciplinary service delivery in school environments: Some limitations. *Physical and Occupational Therapy in Pediatrics* 3(4):9-16.

Ottenbacher, K., and M. Short. 1985. *Vestibular Processing Dysfunction in Children.* New York: The Haworth Press, Inc.

Salek, B., M. A. Braun, M. M. Palmer, and B. Salek. 1983. *Early Detection and Treatment of the Infant and Young Child with Neuromuscular Disorders.* New York: Therapeutic Media, Inc.

Scherzer, A., and I. Tscharnuter. 1982. *Early Diagnosis and Therapy in Cerebral Palsy.* New York: Marcel Dekker, Inc.

Sirvis, B. 1978. Developing IEPs for physically handicapped students: A transdisciplinary viewpoint. *Teaching Exceptional Children* 10(3):78-82.

West, J. F., and L. Adol. 1987. School consultation (Part I): An interdisciplinary perspective on theory, models, and research. *Journal of Learning Disabilities* 20(7):388-408.